For my son, Christoph-Alexander
And for Christine...

"An invasion of armies can be resisted,
but not an idea whose time has come."

———◇———

VICTOR HUGO, 1802–1885
FRENCH POET

Fall

———○———

The leaves are falling, falling as from high above,
Distant gardens fade.
Fall in denying mien.

And in the nights the stolid earth is falling,
Into the loneliness, away from all the stars.

We all shall fall. This hand will fall.
Behold – and so will all the others.

And yet – there is a Someone in whose hands
All our falling rests in boundless gentleness.

———○———

Rainer Maria Rilke, 1875–1926
German Lyric Poet
(Translation by R. Langer)

He Wishes for the Cloths of Heaven

———o———

Had I the heavens' embroidered cloths,
Enwrought with golden and silver light,
The blue and the dim and the dark cloths
Of night and light and the half-light,
I would spread the cloths under your feet:
But I, being poor, have only my dreams;
I have spread my dreams under your feet:
Tread softly because you tread on my dreams.

———o———

WILLIAM BUTLER YEATS, 1865–1939
IRISH LYRIC POET

"There are moments when time does stop.
We must be alert enough to notice such moments."

———○———

JOHN IRVING, A WIDOW FOR ONE YEAR, 1998

Acknowledgements

This book would never have materialized without the help of my friends – friends who have been not just my fellow travellers in the past six years, but have meant much more: shared work, joy, laughter, sorrow, love. Each one of these friends has contributed to this "story of science and research" – and each and every one of them has been and still is important.

First and foremost, thanks are owed to Sentia Faulstich and Thomas Hoppert – as well as all those co-workers and collaborators from the beginning, those early years in my Department of Thoracic and Cardiovascular Surgery in Fulda, Germany. They are my fellow travellers still.

Special thanks to my friend Daniel C. Montano – who so casually midwifed the idea for this book high above the clouds during a flight from Asia to the USA – for making me work so very hard to turn his thoughts into a reality which you now hold in your hands. Ernie Montano, Dan's brother, also brought such fun and warmth into our lives, making my work so much easier. Thank you, Ernie!

My English-Scottish friends, Christine and Grant Gordon, have been good company for so many years.

I count myself lucky to have gained so many friends within the USA – they have supported me with true enthusiasm and open-mindedness, generously contributing their knowledge and experience. Thank you, Judy Pelton, Jack Jacobs, Ralph Bradshaw, and Elizabeth Gordon. And, lately, also Lynne E. Wagoner and Walter H. Merrill of the University of Cincinnati. They have trusted the results of my research and have successfully treated the first patients in the USA.

Jody L. Mack has – and still is – there when I need her assistance in any way – she is responsible for "tying up loose ends."

This project – Angiogenesis – also serves as a bridge between the East and the West. I give very special thanks to my friends in Kiev, Ukraine, without whose help we would not be able to produce FGF-1 (and so much more!) in such an elegant manner: Sergiy Buryak, Olga Tikhova, Oleksandr Vozianov, Vitaliy Kordyum, Irina Slavchenko, and Svetlana Chernukh (who, at the time I write these notes, are experiencing a – hopefully peaceful – revolution in their beautiful country).

Renate Langer has tackled the cause of relieving my English text of any shortcomings with true dedication and enthusiasm. She is responsible for ensuring "ease of reading," and a better understanding of this work.

My thanks go to Matt Jones and Eric Shapiro for the "final finish" of the text and the layout of the end product.

I am grateful to you all.

This book shares the story – my story – of an idea: its course, development, and entrance into reality, between 1992 and 2004.

And the story is not yet at its end – like all great tales, it shall carry on ...

Thomas J. Stegmann
Christmas 2004

For information, about obtaining permission to
reprint material from New Vessels For The Heart,
send your requests by mail (see address below),
email (jmack@cvge.com) or Fax (702-617-5651).

Book Design by Matt Jones (mjones@matthewjstudio.com)
Ghostwritten by Eric Shapiro (USAspeechwriter@aol.com)

Library of Congress Control Number: 2005921193

Stegmann, Thomas Joseph, 1946-
    New Vessels For The Heart / Thomas J. Stegmann. – 1st Edition

    1. Self –publishing 2. Publishers and Publishing.
1. New Vessels For The Heart
Includes bibliographical references and index.
    ISBN: 0-976558-30-5

New Vessels For The Heart is a new version.

Published by CardioVascular BioTherapeutics, Incorporated.
1700 West Horizon Ridge Parkway, Suite #100
Henderson, Nevada 89012
www.cvbt.com

New Vessels for the Heart

———o———

Angiogenesis as New Treatment for
Coronary Heart Disease:

The Story of its Discovery
and Development.

BY THOMAS J. STEGMANN, MD

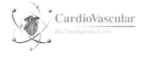

CardioVascular
BioTherapeutics, Inc.

Preface

"Every journey begins with a single step."

This is one of the oldest sayings I know, and it was told to me by my father on almost every day of my childhood. Many people have been told these words. However, my father had his own amendment: "... and a wise man prepares for months before he takes that first step, because every journey is an adventure." His guidance helped me prepare for life and its many journeys. When I met Dr. Thomas Stegmann in 1998, I was very impressed by the journey he was taking in medicine. As I studied what he had accomplished in discovering and advancing the utilization of human proteins – to trigger the natural human healing process in the human heart and treat heart disease – I was amazed.

As the years have passed and I have learned more about this man and his science, I have become more and more astonished. This astonishment led me to ask Dr. Stegmann to ("please") write the story of his discovery of medical angiogenesis and his painstaking work to advance it, despite many obstacles. Building on this train of thought, I have also asked him to look into the future, to speculate on how and where this medical science could evolve.

The book you are holding contains the answers.

This is a book about a journey into a new area of medicine and medical treatment that could affect the lives of millions and millions of people. You will follow the first steps taken by Dr. Stegmann in 1992, his advancements in 1994, his exploration into new frontiers in 1999, and his embrace of new areas of development in 2003. However, this book is not, nor will it ever be, finished. The journey Dr. Stegmann is on gains new advocates every day, and is gathering more researchers to advance its central medical possibility. Medical doctors who grasp the concept are contributing ideas, thoughts, concerns, and guidance every day to illuminate how this new area of medicine can elevate human life.

Originally Dr. Stegmann, as a cardiovascular surgeon, had focused his efforts on growing new blood vessels around clogged arteries in the human heart, to treat a deadly disease known as Coronary Artery Disease. I have watched as the medical clinical trials have proceeded in Germany, and now in the United States. I have watched Dr. Stegmann meet with other medical doctors and researchers to discuss and determine how to progress this medical science to treat Peripheral Vascular Disease, stroke victims, Lumbar Ischemia, wounds, Neurological Diseases, kidneys, bones and ligaments, and much more. I have seen Dr. Stegmann meeting and searching with medical and scientific philosophers in Japan, South Korea, Taiwan, Hong Kong, Thailand, The United Arab Emirates, Saudi Arabia, Greece, the United Kingdom, France, Switzerland, and every part of the United States. In six short years, I have witnessed Dr. Stegmann's efforts to expand this potential medical landmark to a countless number of people.

This book on medical angiogenesis is a brief history of the journey Dr. Stegmann started in 1992. What the book does not tell you is how true my father's words were. Dr. Stegmann's first steps were far more meticulous than anyone can imagine. He prepared for the first step he made in 1992 for years and years. The study of science, medicine, and biology all contributed to preparing Dr. Stegmann for his first step on this journey; however, I believe his prior studies on life, philosophy, morality, self-discipline, and personal courage were even more important. I have repeatedly witnessed the tasks facing Dr. Stegmann, and they were overwhelming. Most people would have surrendered to inertia. Not Dr. Thomas Stegmann; surrendering to mediocrity is not something he can do. If trapped in a perceivable dead end, he would triple his efforts, sacrifice whatever was needed, overcome all obstacles, and end up advancing the medical science another step.

Dr. Stegmann prides himself on being a sailor, and a Baltic Sea sailor at that. Someone who, with great intent, goes into that cold rough sea riding on a wooden stick is someone I do not fully understand. At first I could not imagine the concept of doing this for fun. Then I witnessed the character of this man.

I saw how when the seas of discovery became rough, he sailed though them. I saw when the winds of opinion blew against him, he changed course in order to advance against the winds' force. I saw how when food and water were low, he did without. Finally, I saw how when all about him were in a panic; he calmly took command and saved the day, again, and again, and again.

This book is about his journey. Dr. Stegmann started with discovery, then progressed to advancement, and finally reached a comprehensive understanding of medical angiogenesis. This is a book which I do not believe will be finished in my lifetime. I believe a new, updated version will be needed every few years to report on the advancements. I believe Dr. Stegmann, via his honest and open enquiry into medical angiogenesis, will open the discussion for medical treatments which will change the lives of an infinite number of people.

This is your first step on a journey of understanding what was found, where it stands now, and where it could possibly lead human life.

You are prepared for this journey, because you seek to understand, and that is wonderful.

We all owe a debt of gratitude to Dr. Stegmann for his courage to press forward in a rough and dangerous sea of medical discovery. I remember this quote: "A ship is safe when it is in the harbor; however, that is not what ships were built for." I am sure that Dr. Stegmann had a comfortable and secure life as the head of cardiovascular surgery for a major German hospital. I am sure that he was respected and stable within the traditional medical establishment. Dr. Stegmann left that safe harbor and set sail for what I believe will become one of the great medical journeys of our times. I know he is prepared for this journey, and I know he is a very capable captain. This ship shall reach its destiny.

Most importantly, I – like you – am proud to be a part of this adventure. People I have never met before hug me and thank me for helping to save the lives of their mothers, fathers, and brothers. Letters come in from children, thanking us for saving their mothers' lives.

A day does not go by without my feeling I have done something good. Each of you shares this with me, and with Dr. Stegmann. We are making a difference in the lives of many people every time we take another step in this new area of medicine.

Thank you for your ideas, thoughts, and support. I know you will find Dr. Stegmann's book compelling and informative.

And so we take our first single step ...

Daniel C. Montano
Christmas 2004

*"Discovery is seeing what everyone has seen,
and thinking what no one has thought."*

ALBERT SZENT-GYÖRGYI, 1893–1986
SCIENTIST, NOBEL LAUREATE, 1937

Section I: The Idea

1: The Operating Room

These pages will take you on a journey – back to the beginning, when Angiogenesis as a new treatment for Coronary Heart Disease (CHD) was but a fleeting thought – a bright flicker in my mind. This trip will be an exciting one – for you and for me.

It was a routine operation on a routine day for me and my team. We resided within the walls of the Department of Thoracic & Cardiovascular Surgery – a Department of the Medical Center Fulda, Germany (a 1,000-bed Teaching Hospital, affiliated with the University of Marburg).

Friday, July 17th, 1992. Operating Room 9 – one of the two ORs of the Department of Thoracic & Cardiovascular Surgery:

A male patient, G.S., age 49, father of three children, lies on the operating table. My team has taken care of the preparatory work: the patient's chest is open, and the heart-lung machine is installed and running when I join the operating team. "Basically a straightforward case," I inform my two assistants, "triple-vessel disease. The patient needs three bypass grafts.

The Operating Room   1

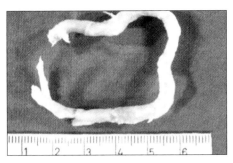 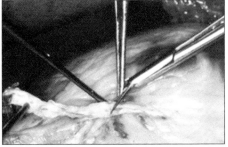

FIGURE 1: The reality of Coronary Artery Disease. **LEFT:** Calcified specimen of right human cornary artery (RCA). **RIGHT:** Surgical procedure of a thrombendarterectomy of the left anterior descending coronary artery (LAD).

The preoperative coronary angiogram also shows diffuse alterations and calcifications of the vascular periphery – besides stenoses of the proximal segments of LAD [i.e., *left anterior descending coronary artery*], CX [i.e., *circumflex artery*], and RCA [i.e., *right coronary artery*]. As if that is not enough, there is a complete occlusion of the distal third of the LAD – bad prognosis. This patient really wants to see how good we are. We have no other choice but to perform three peripheral anastomoses."

Indeed, that's the way it was – the information was correct. The patient showed the expected generalized atherosclerosis of his entire coronary artery system with calcified segments of all coronary arteries, running

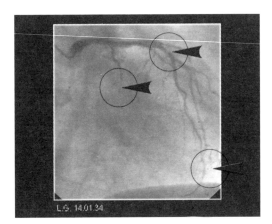

FIGURE 2:

Coronary angiogram (left coronary artery) demonstrating diffuse Coronary Artery Disease, also affecting proximal artery segments as the periphery (arrows) of the entire coronary artery system.

down from the proximal parts of the LCA (i.e., *left coronary artery*) and RCA to the periphery of the side branches (diagonal, marginal, posterolateral); the LAD was particularly calcified, heavily, down to the apex of the left ventricle. I performed a triple aorto-coronary bypass grafting – using the left IMA (i.e., *internal mammary artery*) for the LAD, the right IMA for the RCA, and a vein graft for the main and largest marginal branch of the CX. The weaning off the pump was successful. After the routine insertion of chest tubes and the closure of the sternum and cutis, the patient was transferred from the OR to the ICU. Eight days later, G.S. left the Medical Center Fulda after an uneventful postoperative recovery period.

Walking back from the OR to my office, I reflected on the operation, the intraoperative details, and both the particulars and the prognosis of the patient. Suddenly, I remembered an article I had read some days earlier. The article, published by *J. Folkman's* group, dealt with tumour growth, and with ways to stop that growth while treating cancer. The so-called *"growth factors,"* particularly those with angiogenic potency, played a very important role in tumour growth processes. Tumour researchers were trying to both stop and block those angiogenic growth factors, hoping to reduce a given tumour's size by reducing or destroying its vasculature ...

"Yes," I thought to myself, "what an interesting idea – I like their approach to THEIR problem. We, however, should attack our problem from another angle. What the tumour researchers do not want (growth of the vascular system), would be very much desired by OUR patients that suffer from narrowed, calcified, occluded vessels (Figure 1, Figure 2)! This would provide them with new vessels and arteries, replacing the old, destroyed original coronary arteries ... We have to start researching these options. That would really be a boon to heart patients. It could prolong their lives – but not just prolong them, imbue them with excitement and possibilities! In the long run, it could also save them and their health insurance providers – actually, the entire healthcare system! – quite a lot of money. These people would be able to go back to work again sooner, and their working lives would be extended. And as their working lives were prolonged – they would get a whole new lease on life ..."

My mind was running on overtime.

"The blood more stirs
To rouse a lion than to start a hare!"

These lines from Shakespeare's *King Henry IV* rushed through my head – I wanted my patients to live like lions, not hares. I wanted them to enjoy life to the fullest, and I would stop at nothing to make this possible.

2: The Background of Coronary Heart Disease (CHD)

Atherosclerosis, or Cardiovascular Disease (CVD), is universally present to some degree in all adults, and clinically manifests as Coronary Heart Disease (CHD), cerebrovascular disease, and Peripheral Vascular Disease (PVD). The Framingham Study has demonstrated that the lifetime risk of developing CHD, the most common and most lethal of cardiovascular diseases, at the age of 40 years is 49 percent for men and 32 percent for women. About 20 million members (or 8 percent) of the US population have some form of heart disease. About 4.4 million US adults (2 percent of the population) have had strokes, and approximately one in four stroke victims are restricted from their usual day-to-day activities.

According to the AHA (2004 Update), one in five males and females in the US has some form of Cardiovascular Disease (CVD). 13.2 million Americans suffer from Coronary Heart Disease (CHD), 7.8 million per year experience heart attacks (myocardial infarction), and 6.8 million have angina pectoris (chest pains). Nearly 2,600 Americans die of CVD each day, an average of one death every 34 seconds. CVD claims more lives each year than the next 5 leading causes of death combined – cancer, chronic lower respiratory diseases, accidents, diabetes mellitus, and influenza and pneumonia.

This year (2004) an estimated 700,000 Americans will have a new coronary attack (Figure 3). About 500,000 will have recurrent attacks. The average age of a person having a first heart attack is 65.8 for men and 70.4 for women. CHD is the single largest killer of American males and females. About every 26 seconds, an American will suffer a coronary event, and about every minute, someone will die from one. About 42 percent of those who experience coronary attacks in a given year will die from them.

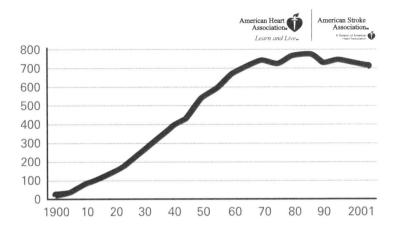

FIGURE 3: Deaths from diseases of the heart: USA 1900–2001. AHA update 2004.

From 1979 to 2001, the number of Americans discharged from short-stay hospitals with CHD as the first-listed diagnosis increased by 27 percent (Figure 4). Equally interesting is the fact that the estimated direct and indirect cost of CHD in 2004 was $133.2 billion (Figure 5).

The major modifiable risk factors contributing to the occurrence of atherosclerotic diseases remain highly prevalent. Despite a decline in cigarette smoking over the last 30 years, 49 million Americans (one in four adults) still smoke. The average plasma total cholesterol has decreased significantly, but more than half of all adults – 98 million – have cholesterol levels exceeding 200 mg/dl, and of these 39 million have levels of over 240 mg/dl. The treatment and control of hypertension has improved substantially since 1970, but 50 million Americans still suffer from it today.

Alarmingly, obesity and diabetes are on the rise. One third of our adults are now overweight (>25 kg/m2), while approximately 10 million

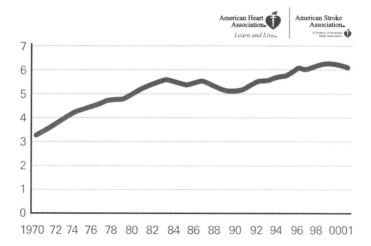

American Heart Association.
Learn and Live.

American Stroke Association.
A Division of American Heart Association

FIGURE 4: Hospital discharges for cardiovascular diseases: USA 1970–2001. AHA update 2004.

Americans are currently at a greatly increased risk of atherosclerotic cardiovascular events because they have diabetes. Diabetes and obesity are now beginning to be regarded as features of an insulin-resistance syndrome comprised of glucose intolerance, abdominal obesity, dyslipidemia, elevated blood pressure, and hyperinsulinemia.

Both type 1 and type 2 Diabetes are associated with accelerated-atherogenesis that accounts for most of the mortality among diabetics. In both types of diabetes, microvascular sequelae such as retinopathy and nephropathy appear to be related to glucose control, although most type 2 diabetics have an insulin resistance syndrome. The risk of macrovascular disease in diabetics is greater when accompanied by any of the often associated risk factors. Diabetes escalates the risk associated with any of the prevalent cardiovascular risk factors.

The situation pertaining to Asian Indians is a special and rather unique one. Asian Indians, wherever they live, have the highest rate of CAD despite the fact that nearly half of them are lifelong vegetarians. The CAD death rates among overseas Asian Indians have been 50 percent to 300 percent higher than those of American, European, Chinese, and Japanese people, irrespective of gender, religion, or social class. Among those below 30, the CAD mortality rate among Asian Indians is 3 times higher than that of Caucasians in the United Kingdom, and 10 times higher than that of Chinese residents of Singapore.

During the past three decades, the average age of first-time heart attack patients has increased by 10 years in the US, but decreased by 10 years in India. About 50 percent of all heart attacks among Asian Indian men occur when they are under the age of 55, and 25 percent when they are under the age of 40.

3: Existing Treatments Available for CHD

To this day, there are various forms of treatment for Coronary Artery Disease in widespread use in the US as well as in highly developed, industrialized countries throughout the world (Figure 5). These include:

1. Drugs: particularly nitrates, beta blocking drugs, calcium-channel-blocking agents, lipid lowering drugs, ACE-inhibiting drugs, Aspirin.

2. Interventional procedures: namely PTCA (Angioplasty), insertion of stents (it is presently very common to use so-called "drug eluting stents").

3. Coronary Artery Bypass Surgery (CABG).

According to the AHA, 1,051,000 angioplasty procedures, 516,000 bypass procedures (CABG), 1,314,000 diagnostic cardiac catheterizations, 46,000 implantable defibrillators, and 177,000 pacemaker procedures are performed annually in the US (based on 2001 figures).

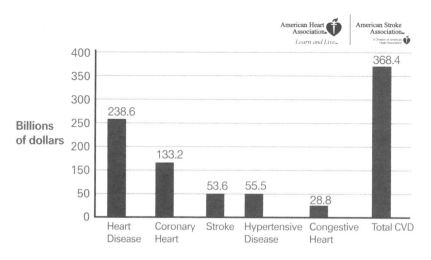

FIGURE 5: Costs of cardiovascular diseases and stroke: USA 2004. AHA update 2004.

4: Angiogenic Growth Factors

A broad variety of so-called "growth factors" exist which are able to stimulate and/or initiate neovascularization via stimulation of endothelial cell proliferation and migration. These are called *"angiogenic growth factors"* – and all of them are proteins (poly-peptides). In addition, effects such as stimulation of extracellular matrix breakdown, attraction of pericytes amd macrophages, stimulation of smooth muscle cell proliferation and migration, formation of new vascular structures, and the deposition of new matrix are part of the biological process initiated and guided by angiogenic growth factors.

Today we know from extensive experimental research that the following growth factors have the potential to stimulate vessel growth:

- Fibroblast Growth Factor (FGF)
- Granulocyte Colony Stimulating Factor (G-CSF)
- Hepatocyte Growth Factor (HGF)
- Interleukin-8 (IL-8)
- Placental Growth Factor (PGF)
- Platelet-Derived Endothelial Cell Growth Factor (PD-ECGF)
- Platelet-Derived Growth Factor (PDGF)
- Transforming Growth Factor-alpha (TGF-alpha)
- Transforming Growth Factor-beta (TGF-beta)
- Tumor Necrosis Factor-alpha (TNF-alpha)
- Vascular Endothelial Growth Factor (VEGF)

In particular, the various members of the FGF-family stimulate the proliferation of mesodermal cells and many cells of neuroectodermal, ectodermal, and endodermal origin. So far, the members of the FGF-family seem to have the most effective potency regarding the induction of neo-angiogenesis. In addition, FGF-1 (and FGF-2) is particularly very active as a potent regulator in nerve regeneration, cartilage repair, and wound healing.

5: Fibroblast Growth Factor (FGF)

Fibroblast Growth Factors (FGFs) represent a large family of polypeptides that are potent regulators of cell growth and differentiation (Figure 6). They play a major role in normal embryonic development, and in tissue repair and regeneration. FGFs act on cells that are primarily of mesodermal origin, but also have broader effects on cells derived from the ectoderm and endoderm. Depending on the target cell, the conditions of cell culture, and the presence or absence of other trophic agents, FGFs alter migration, morphology, differentiation, and proliferation. Though first discovered for their impact on fibroblasts, hence their name, their activities and physiological roles are considerably more extensive than is implied by that name. In fact, some members of the FGF family are not even mitogens for fibroblasts at all, and would be understood far better if thought of as epithelial growth factors.

The FGFs comprise a group of structurally similar polypeptides which currently includes 22 different members (FGF-1 to FGF-22). The first members of this family, FGF-1 (acidic FGF, aFGF) and FGF-2 (basic FGF,

Fibroblast Growth Factor 1 (FGF-1)

- FGF family contains 22 members
- 4 Different receptors in FGF family
- FGF-1 alone interacts with all 4 receptors
- FGF-1 promotes both angiogenesis and arteriogenesis

FIGURE 6:   Fibroblast Growth Factor-1: Details.

b-FGF) were described in 1986. All members of the FGF-family range in molecular weight from 17 to 34 kDa in vertebrates, and some of them are glycosylated (Figure 7). FGFs have been shown to interact with three different types of binding partners: heparin suphate proteoglycans, a cysteine-rich transmembrane FGF-binding protein (which appears to be involved in the regulation of intracellular FGF trafficking), and *four high-affinity transmembrane FGF receptors of the tyrosine kinase* family, which are responsible for signal transduction.

The FGF-receptors, *FGFR-1 to FGFR-4,* are transmembrane protein tyrosine kinases with either two or three immunoglobulin-like domains or a heparin binding sequence in the extracellular part of the receptor. Most of the FGFs bind to a specific subset of FGF-receptors, *FGF-1, however, binds to all (four) receptors* (Figure 6).

A characteristic feature of FGFs is their interaction with heparin or heparin sulphate proteoglycans. These interactions stabilize FGFs and may limit their diffusion and release into interstitial spaces. Most importantly, the interaction of FGFs with heparin or heparin sulphate proteoglycans is essential for the activation of the signalling receptor (Figure 8).

FGFs and their receptors are expressed at multiple sites in both the developing and adult organism, which underscores the important role of FGFs in development and tissue homeostasis. This hypothesis has been confirmed by the wide variety of phenotypic abnormalities observed in FGF and FGFR knockout animals.

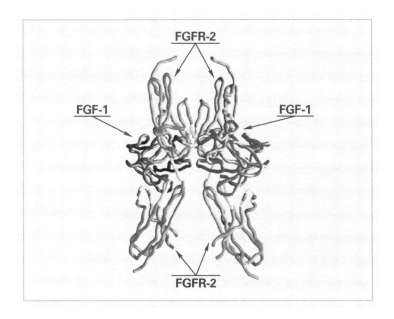

FIGURE 7: Three-dimensional model of the structure of FGF-1 and receptors (FGFR-2).

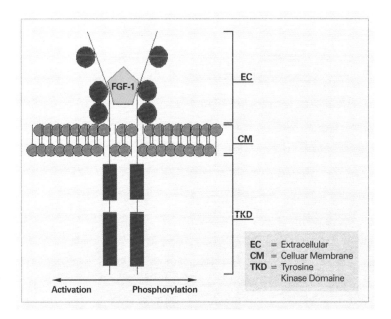

FIGURE 8: Interaction of FGF-1 with the cell surface (cell membrane).

EC = Extracellular space   CM = Cell membrane
TKD = Tyrosine Kinase Domain

6: The Principle of Angiogenesis

Therapeutic angiogenesis can be defined, broadly, as the use biological agents, bioactive materials, or environmental conditions to stimulate the growth of new blood vessels, to restore or augment the circulatory perfusion of tissues, to reverse ischemia, or to accelerate healing. Accordingly, this approach has been developed for the treatment of ischemic heart disease, cerebrovascular disease, critical limb ischemia, and delayed wound healing.

Inside of established blood vessels within mature organisms, the endothelial cells remain in a quiescent, non-proliferative state until the stimulation of angiogenesis occurs via conditions such as wounding, inflammation, hypoxia, or ischemia. The formation of new vessels is the result of several processes: dissolution of the matrix underlying the endothelial cell line; migration, adhesion, and proliferation of endothelial cells; and formation of a new three-dimensional tube, which then lengthens from its tip as circulation is re-established. For larger vessels, vascular smooth muscle cells migrate as well, and adhere to the newly deposited matrix of the nascent vessel. Angiogenic growth factors induce, promote, or interfere with all these steps of angiogenesis.

In addition to their role in the initial development of the vascular system, angiogenic growth factors – like FGF and VEGF – and their receptors are expressed by endothelial cells in capillaries sprouting from established vessels in response to pathological conditions. The expression of receptors for FGF and VEGF varies according to the vascular bed, with little or no expression present in the normal myocardium, and can be altered by ischemia. Reduction of oxygen tension promotes enhanced expression

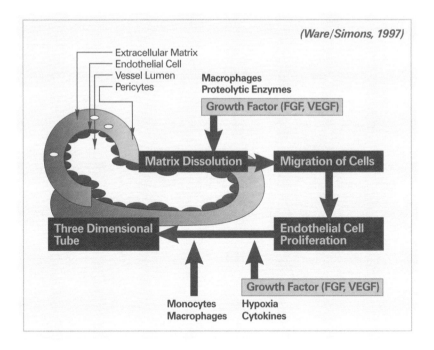

FIGURE 9:   Principle of induction of angiogenesis.

FGF = Fibroblast Growth Factor
VEGF = Vascular Endothelial Growth Factor

of mitogens, including FGF, VEGF, PDGF, and their receptors, as well as endothelial cell growth.

Also important for any effect of growth factors, particularly FGF, is the binding system on the surface of the cell membrane (Figure 9). Though various forms of FGF-Receptors (FGFRs) exist, the basic structure of all FGFRs is the same: they belong to the immunoglobulin (Ig)-like family of tyrosin kinases. The FGF ligand-FGF receptor interaction is complicated by the role played by proteoglycans in FGF action. Specifically, FGFs have an unusually high affinity for heparin sulfates, which translates into an ability to interact with glycosaminoglycanes like heparin. This binding causes conformational changes in the FGFs, which result in altered receptor binding and protect the ligand from proteolysis and acid degeneration. Most importantly, this interaction appears to be required for significant ligand-receptor binding. Extracellular FGF binds to heparin sulphate proteoglycans in the matrix and at the cell surface, so this binding is believed to both protect the FGFs and serve as a reservoir of FGFs that are available after trauma, injury, or any pathophysiological event that might require a rapid mobilization of FGF activity (like angiogenesis).

And so the idea was born – but how and where to start with the research, the tests? The efficacy of FGF-1 needed to be shown, and (this was a top priority to me) any eventual negative side effects of the growth factor had to be excluded.

The research was to occur in two steps:

1. **Laboratory tests with cell cultures in order to prove the efficacy of FGF-1.**

2. **Animal experiments**

As it turned out, producing the FGF-1 made for a very complex and time-consuming procedure (see Chapter 7). The research and testing would take a long time – much longer than was originally anticipated. It was going to be a very long journey indeed.

With so many tests to run, some small setbacks were inevitable – but I was certain that I was on the right road to finding another, less invasive method for helping heart patients return to good health. In fact, it would take me roughly three years until I was ready to apply for the patent. I persevered, and in the end I would be proven right. All the while, I kept the words of one Benjamin Disraeli (1804–1616) in mind:

"The secret of success is never to lose sight of your goal."

Though I was certain of my goal – to help patients avoid extensive surgery; to aid stroke victims and diabetics – my research would produce more possibilities for FGF-1 than I'd originally thought possible.

> *"What is the highest level of human happiness?*
> *To do what we understand as right and good."*

Johann Wolfgang von Goethe, 1749–1832
German Poet and Philosopher

Section II: Pre-Clinical Research

7: Production of FGF-1

Apathogenic strains of E. coli were genetically manipulated (35 bacterial cultures) so as to produce human FGF-1. A plasmid which carried genetic information for the production of human FGF-1 was introduced into the microorganism. Following centrifugation and ultrasonic treatment and mixture with inductors and enzymes, the elution of FGF-1 was carried out by heparin-sepharose column adsorption chromatography. Thus, each of several elution fractions with particular elution buffer molarity were collected and purified by dialysis. In addition, various tests were applied to ensure that the isolated substances were indeed FGF-1. Elution fractions showing positive proof of protein content were characterized by BIO-RAD assay via 11.25 percent sodium dodecyl sulphate polyacrylamide (SDS) electrophoresis. Biochemical isolation of the FGF-1 was also confirmed by qualitative testing for the corresponding antigen structure by Western blot analysis. The IgG antibody put in use originated in the Laboratory of Molecular Biology in Rockville, USA. At the end of the procedure an additional — and in our opinion, decisive — purification of the growth factor obtained was carried out via high-pressure liquid chromatography (HPLC). The method for this was based upon the procedure of *Gospodarowicz*. Only those elution fractions that had been proved by BIO-RAD protein determination and SDS electrophoresis to contain FGF-1 were submitted to HPLC purification. The factors purified in this manner were then lyophilised and stored at −32 °C.

We were able to extract the human growth factor FGF-1 from all 35 bacterial cultures. It was possible to establish the presence of FGF-1 qualitatively via SDS electrophoresis in all of the complete elution fractions showing positive proof of their protein nature by way of the BIO-RAD assay (average 60 µg±7 µg per 100 ml eluate).

After this qualitative assessment, the samples were purified further using high-pressure fluid chromatography (HPLC). This process makes it possible to eliminate remaining impurities such as *E. coli* proteins, and to extract the isolated growth factor FGF-1 after a running time of 70 minutes. The antigen structure of the highly purified factor obtained in this way was established in all of these samples using Western blot analysis.

8: Cell Culture Experiments

For the endothelial cell culture, 40 segments of the great saphenous vein were routinely removed in the operating room during the course of aorto-coronary bypass operations.

Endothelial cells from all the venous segments were cultured successfully. Following their removal from the vein, the initial cell density in the cultures was about 2.6 x l04 cells per cm2. From a total of 189 cell cultures, three groups were generated: group 1 (control) contained 49 cultures, and groups 2 (FGF-1) and 3 (FGF-1 plus 1.0 mg heparin) contained 70 cultures each. FGF-1 was added in various concentrations to group 2 and group 3: 0.02; 0.1; 0.2; 1.0; 2.0; 10.0; 20.0 ng per ml cell suspension (10 cultures each). Confluent monolayers developed in all these cultures: after 8 to 11 days in group 1, and after 5 to 8 days in group 2 (with growth factor) and group 3 (with growth factor plus heparin).

In addition, the number of endothelial cells in all three groups was measured with a cell-counter. We found the largest number of cells in group 3 after the administration of 0.2 ng FGF-1/ml medium (8.l x 104 EC/ml medium). Without the addition of heparin (group 2), a maximum count of only 5.8 x 104 EC/ml medium was achieved.

Measurement of the inclusion of tritium and thymidine showed a significant increase ($p < 0.005$) in the rate of DNA synthesis in cultures to which FGF-1 had been added (groups 2 and 3). The addition of heparin to the culture medium produced a further significant rise in this effect: group 1 compared with group 2: 0.02 ng; 10.0 ng: 20.0 ng per ml FGF-1 ($p < 0.01$); group 2 compared with group 3: 0.1 ng; 0.2 ng, 1.0 ng; 2.0 ng per ml FGF-1 ($p < 0.005$).

The influence of FGF-1 on endothelial cell cultures

Segments of the human great saphenous vein removed in the course of a bypass operation were used for the isolation and culture of endothelial cells via the method described by *Watkins et al.* Three separate groups of endothelial cell cultures were investigated and compared with one another (see above). One group served as a control. FGF-1 was added to the other two groups in concentrations of 0.02, 0.1, 0.2, 1.0, 2.0, 10 or 20 ng/ml cell suspension – in one case with and in the other without the addition of 1.0 mg/ml heparin. The endothelial cells were cultured as far as the development of the first complete monolayer, and the number of cells in all three groups counted with a cell-counter. Confluent monolayers developed in all these cultures; after 8 to 11 days in group 1, and after 5 to 8 days in group 2 (with growth factor) and group 3 (with growth factor plus heparin).

The mitogenic action of FGF-1 (with and without heparin) on the endothelial cells was evaluated not only by cell counting but also by measuring the rate of DNA synthesis in the cells. The cell cultures were obtained as described above, and the rate of DNA synthesis determined by *Klagsbrun's* method. Measurement of the inclusion of tritium and thymidine showed a significant increase ($p < 0.005$) in the rate of DNA synthesis in cultures to which FGF-1 had been added (groups 2 and 3). The addition of heparin to the culture medium produced a further significant rise in this effect: group 1 compared with group 2: 0.02 ng; 10.0 ng: 20.0 ng per ml FGF-1 ($p < 0.01$); group 2 compared with group 3: 0.1 ng; 0.2 ng, 1.0 ng; 2.0 ng per ml FGF-1 ($p < 0.005$).

Chorioallantoic membrane assay

In order to investigate the angiogenic action of the growth factor *in vivo*, the established method of Chorioallantoic Membrane

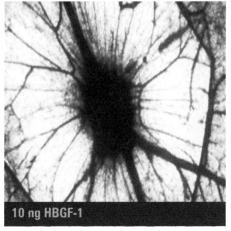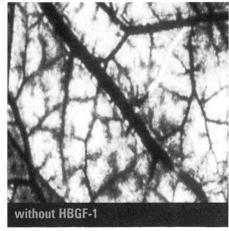

10 ng HBGF-1

without HBGF-1

FIGURE 10: Chorion-Allantois-Membrane Assay (CAM): **LEFT**: Neovascularization after application of 10 ng FGF-1. **RIGHT**: Control.

HBGF-1 = Heparin-Binding Growth Factor-1 = **FGF-1**

Assay (CMA) was employed. This made it possible to demonstrate the immediate influence of growth factors on living tissue, since the growth of the membrane on capillary systems can be observed directly under a light microscope. Fertilised hens' eggs were incubated for 13 days. The growth factor was then added to the membrane, and the specimens covered with Thermanox tissue-culture coverslips. The membrane was examined with a light microscope (magnification x 1O) after 4 days, so that a direct comparison between membranes with and without the addition of FGF-1 could be made. A control group was treated with heat-denatured (70°C for three minutes) FGF-1.

The light microscopic evaluation of the chorioallantoic membrane assay took place on the 4th day, after the growth factor FGF-1 – or, in the case of the control group, of the denatured FGF-1 – was administered. Whereas in the normal physiologically developed chorioallantoic membrane only a weak, net-like arrangement of the structures could be witnessed using the light microscope, in the regions of the membrane incubated with

FGF-1, the sprouting of extra-capillary structures could be clearly seen. In this case, the essential criterion for the recognition of new structures was their radial orientation outwards from each site of application (Figure 10).

The light microscopic picture of the CAM revealed a significant increase in the appearance of blood vessels in the membrane following the administration of FGF-1, compared to the control group, which had received only the heat-denatured FGF-1. In the latter group, nothing inconsistent with the normal developmental stages was found. In this way it was possible to verify the development of new vessels in the CAM after the administration of FGF-1, and thus confirm the angiogenic potential of this substance with a simple biological test.

These results were very encouraging to me. It was a *premiere* – the first time that the growth of new vessels was observed in living tissue following administration of a low dose of FGF-1. At long last, I had seen a visible confirmation of what I'd been certain FGF-1 could do all along.

The preparation for and realization of these tests was very time-consuming, which was at times quite frustrating for me. I wanted to move on to the animal experiments, wanted to collect the necessary data to ascertain that I was, indeed, on the right path – that I was on my way to reaching the goal I'd set.

9: Animal Experiments

Exclusion of pyrogenic effects of FGF-1 in animal experiments

In order to exclude any pyrogenic effects of the growth factor, various concentrations (0.01, 0.5 and 1.0 mg/kg) of FGF-1 were injected subcutaneously, intramuscularly, or intravenously into a total of 27 white New Zealand rabbits. To serve as controls, a further 13 animals were given a solution containing only the heat-denatured factor. On the day of injection, rectal temperatures were taken at half-hourly intervals during the first 3 hours, and hourly thereafter. For the following 12 days, temperatures were recorded at intervals of 8 hours.

During the same period, the white cell count, ESR (Erythrocyte Sedimentation Rate), and C-reactive protein were determined daily.

The possible pyrogenicity of the human growth factor FGF-1 could be confidently excluded in an established animal model. In none of the 27 experimental animals –nor in the 13 controls – was there any significant rise in the closely controlled body temperature during the time of the observation, or any indication of the development of an inflammatory reaction. The white cell count, ESR, and C-reactive protein were shown to remain within normal limits via the daily examination of blood taken from an ear vein. This result was independent of both the concentration of the growth factor and its route of injection (i.v., s.c. or i.m.).

Cell cultures and animal experiments exclude the possibility of tumour stimulation by FGF-1

Now, let us take a moment and go back to the start of this journey – the day I remembered the article by *J. Folkman* on how to deal with and ultimately stop tumour growth. FGF-1 was stimulating the growth of new vessels – I wanted to make certain beyond all doubt that FGF-1 would have only positive effects. Although this would, yet again, call for time-consuming additional testing, I insisted on conducting these tests in order to *definitively* exclude a stimulation of tumour growth due to the administration of FGF-1. Naturally, any other negative side effects were to be excluded as well – to finalize testing on animals and to freely apply for the clinical trials.

To exclude the possibility of any oncoproliferative action of the growth factor FGF-1, we carried out stimulation tests on human tumour cell strains. We investigated the following tumours by means of H-thymidine assay: pleomorphic cell sarcoma, hypernephroma, melanoma, and small cell carcinoma of the bronchus. With each strain, the initial cell count amounted to 500 cells per hole in a plate of 96 holes. Stimulation of the tumour-cell cultures was carried out with various concentrations of the factor: group 1 (control group), culture without FGF-1; group 2, culture with 10 ng FGF-1; and group 3, culture with 100 ng FGF-1. The stimulation was allowed to continue for a period totalling 24 hours.

To further exclude the tumour-stimulating action of FGF-1, strains of human tumour cells were implanted into experimental animals (mice). For each tumour, an initial quantity of 3×10^6 cells was implanted subcutaneously. The tumour cells were taken up in 0.1 ml of culture medium and injected subcutaneously into the right side of the abdominal wall of the mouse (unconscious via ether anaesthesia). The experimental animals were divided into four groups for each tumour cell strain. The total number of animals was 320. Group 1 (n = 80) received only tumour cells, group 2 (n = 80) received tumour cells and systemic FGF-1, group 3 (n = 80) received a tumour and growth factor suspension, and group 4 (n = 80) received only the growth factor. The weight of the living animals was measured at intervals of four days. In addition, the TPS (Tissue Polypeptide Specific) for each animal was determined after 6 weeks, and again after 12 weeks.

These experiments continued for 12 weeks. The tumours were explanted and their size and weight measured. They were also assessed histologically.

The stimulation tests carried out on the various strains of human tumour cells enabled us to exclude any possible tumour-stimulating action of the growth factor FGF-1. The results of the ^{3}H-thymidine assay were sufficient to eliminate the possibility of a stimulation of the following human tumour strains: pleomorphic cell sarcoma, hypernephroma, melanoma, and small cell carcinoma of the bronchus. Neither in group 2 (tumour cell cultures plus 10 ng of the factor solution) nor in group 3 (tumour cell culture plus 100 ng of the factor solution) could we find any increase in the rate of DNA synthesis in comparison to the control culture in group 1 (tumour cell culture without FGF-1).

During our experiments on naked mice, histological examination and the determination of the TPS (Tissue Polypeptide Specific) enabled us to exclude the possibility that tumour induction can result from the administration of FGF-1 by itself. It is equally true that neither the local nor systemic introduction of FGF-1 can stimulate tumours already implanted (pleomorphic cell sarcoma, hypernephroma, melanoma, and small cell carcinoma of the bronchus) to increase in either size or malignancy. In neither the size and weight nor the histological grading of the tumours was there any significant difference between the control animals (tumours alone) and the experimental groups with tumours and FGF-1 in varying concentrations.

It was also impossible to find any significant difference between the TPS titre of the control and the experimental animals. In none of the experimental animals which received the growth factor alone did the histology show any tumour, or the serology show any rise in the TPS titre.

The results of these tests were very encouraging. I was relieved and elated – the journey was to go on. I would have liked to speed up the process of trials; there were millions of potential patients waiting for treatment. This growth factor therapy would be able to help *millions of people*. However, there were to be no shortcuts; I would rather spend some more months running tests than go on to the clinical trials with insufficient data. These tests were to show the positive effects of FGF-1 on the animals' vessels. They were designed to prove and make visible the efficacy of FGF-1.

Another series of animal experiments was carried out.

Demonstration of the angiogenic potential of FGF-1 in animal experiments

FGF-1 itself was also investigated in experimental animals. In 12 Lewis inbred rats, the pericardium was carefully divided through a left-sided thoracotomy incision, and a piece of a vascular prosthesis (PTFE = Polytetrafluorethylene), previously treated with 1 µg FGF-1, was inserted

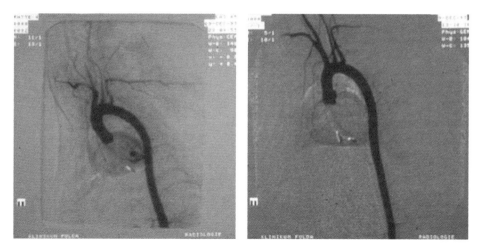

FIGURE 11: Ischemic rat heart experiments. Two clips are marking the experimentally created ischemia in the area of the distal LAD. **LEFT**: Neovascularization after application of 10μ FGF-1. **RIGHT**: Control. HBGF-1 = FGF-1

between the myocardium and the descending aorta. In the control group (n = 6), a similar piece of prosthetic material was implanted which had not been treated.

Thereafter, the impact of FGF-1 on the *ischemic rat heart* was investigated (Figure 11). Rats of the same breed were used (a total of 275 animals; the 125 that did not receive FGF-1 served as the control group). The upper abdomen was opened by a transverse laparotomy incision, the diaphragm was divided, and the pericardium was split at the apex of the heart. Two titanium clips were inserted, clipping the peripheral LAD in order to induce myocardial ischemia. The growth factor was then introduced directly into the myocardium at the edge of the ischemic tissue (average dose: 10 µg). Twelve weeks later, an angiographic examination of the coronary artery system was carried out via aortic root angiography. Finally, the myocardium at the site of the injection of the growth factor was analyzed histologically.

All animals received human care in compliance with the *"Principles of Laboratory Animal Care"* – formulated by the National Society for Medical Research – and the *"Guide for the Care and Use of Laboratory Animals"* – prepared by the National Academy of Sciences and published by the National Institute of Health (NIH Publication No. 85-23, revised 1985).

We examined a total of 275 inbred Lewis rats: 150 experimental animals treated with FGF-1, and 125 control animals. During and shortly after the operation, 14 (9.3 percent) of the experimental animals, and 19 (15.2 percent) of the controls died. During the 12-week period of observation before the angiographic follow-up, an additional 4 (3 percent) experimental animals and 3 (3 percent) controls also died.

We were able to carry out successful aortic root angiography on all the surviving animals by injecting contrast medium into the right common carotid artery through a 24 G catheter. After 12 weeks, amid all the experimental animals in which we had previously induced myocardial ischemia with titanium clips and thereafter administered growth factor directly into the heart muscles, a clearly unambiguous increase in the accumulation of contrast medium in the region of injected growth factor could be recognized angiographically (Figure 11). Owing to the presence of the titanium clips, we were able to perceive the increased accumulation of contrast medium in the transitional zone between the infarcted and the healthy myocardium. On the other hand, in the control group without growth factor application, not one animal showed a similar increased accumulation of the contrast medium.

In the histological picture of the myocardium taken from animals into which growth factor had been injected intramyocardially, numerous new vessels could be detected in sections between the healthy myocardium

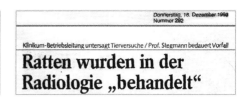

FIGURE 12: Newspaper in Germany I: FZ from December 13, 1993.

FIGURE 13: Newspaper in Germany II: FZ from December 16, 1993.

and the scar tissue of the infarcted area. All these new vessels showed a normal three-layered vessel wall (average: 235 capillaries/mm^2). In none of the control animals could we find either a significant increase in accumulation of contrast medium or a histologically comparable high density of vessels (average: 129 capillaries / mm^2). After evaluating all of the histological findings, we saw that the animals treated with FGF-1 had a significantly higher number of sectioned vessels in comparison to the controls ($p < 0.01$).

Unfortunately, this – scientifically essential! – step in the experiments caused an outcry in the local news media (Figure 12, Figure 13). *Angiography was used on rats in the hospital!* It was a "scandal." The mayor of the city of Fulda criticised me – however I remained unmoved by all these manoeuvres to make me stop my experiments. I explained to the public, the media, why this procedure was so important. I was disappointed to no end that these people were so petty. Not to mention the fact that this research was funded by myself, and supported by a private "not-for-profit" Foundation in Fulda, Germany, which was interested in the progress of any kind of human heart disease treatment. The research was also done on weekends, when other doctors were spending time with their families, attending soccer games, or otherwise relaxing...

A number of those who criticised me then would eventually benefit from the findings (and later, results) of that research (Figure 14). Would they stick to their position once they needed the FGF-1 treatment? As it turned out, once I was lauded by the world press, including the Wall Street Journal, for our findings, the city would have liked nothing better then to have our Company plant its roots in Fulda. However, later on, Dan Montano and I decided to found the Company in the United States.

Summary of Experimental Results

Cell culture - Human venous endothelial cells

- Significant increase of DNA synthesis rate
- Cell counting: Significant increase for FGF-1 plus Heparin
- Confluent monolayer: 5-8 vs. 8-11 days

Animal experiments (non-ischemic)

- Side-directed new vessel growth between descending aorta and left ventricle

Animal experiments (ischemic rat heart)

- Significant increase in # of sectioned vessels:
  235 capillaries/mm^2 (FGF-1)
  129 capillaries/mm^2 (Controls)

FIGURE 14: Summary of the experimental results, Germany 1994: Proof of angiogenic efficacy of FGF-1.

*"While the sick man has life
there is hope."*

MARCUS TULLIUS CICERO, 106–43 B.C.
ROMAN POLITICIAN & PHILOSOPHER

Section III: Human Clinical Trials

10: 1st Human Clinical Trial (1995-1996)

My journey had reached its final stages – *human clinical trials*. Our research on the basic effects of FGF-1 on endothelial cells and cell cultures, as well as the experiments on animals, had taken almost three years. We had been successful in excluding serious negative side effects such as the stimulation of tumour growth due to the administration of FGF-1. We had also been successful in proving the efficacy of FGF-1 in both cell culture experiments and animal experiments.

The next and most important step on my journey to my desired goal was to obtain permission from the Ethics Commission to perform human clinical trials. I decided that I would minimize the risks to patients during the first clinical trial by administering FGF-1 only to those patients already in need of a heart operation, a coronary artery bypass grafting procedure (Figure 15). *Only* those patients whose occluded subsidiary branches of the coronary artery system could not be revascularized surgically were to be treated with FGF-1.

The clinical administration of FGF-1 to patients with Coronary Heart Disease

During extensive preliminary animal experiments, it was possible to obtain convincing evidence for the clear angiogenic potency of growth factor FGF-1 on the ischemic myocardium in animals. Any tumour-stimulating side effect of FGF-1, or pyrogenicity caused by that protein, could similarly be excluded by a large series of experiments. As a consequence of these promising results, we were able to obtain consent from the Ethics Commission of the Philipps-University Marburg, our responsible authority, for the *world's first clinical trial on humans using angiogenic growth factor therapy* (namely those suffering from CHD). The clinical study included 40 patients. All participants were thoroughly informed about the nature and aim of the study, including the risks of additional investigation, and freely formalized their willingness to take part. The patients selected were those for whom, because of their multiple coronary vascular diseases, elective surgical revascularization had already been decided upon. Patients who had already undergone heart surgery, and patients with a history of investigated myocardial infarction and a consequent reduction in the ejection fraction of the left ventricle (EF < 40 percent), were excluded from the beginning. In selecting

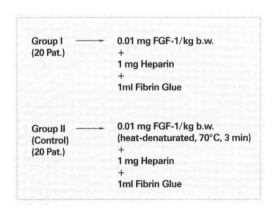

FIGURE 15: First human clinical trial, Germany 1995–1996. Study design.

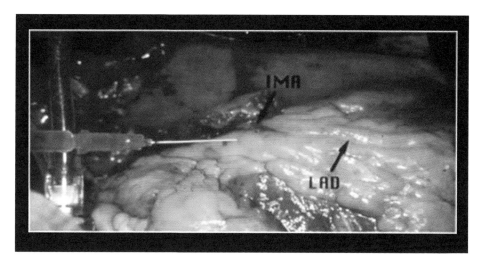

FIGURE 16: First human clinical trial. Intraoperative view: Intramyocardial injection of FGF-1 during CABG-procedure.

IMA = Internal mammary artery
LAD = Left anterior descending coronary artery

participants for the study, particular importance was placed upon patients with comparable coronary morphology. In all cases, there was a high-grade stenosis of the LAD (left anterior descending artery) with a further peripheral stenosis of the vessel itself, or of a subsidiary branch, that could not be revascularized surgically.

In every case, we decided to bridge over the proximal stenosis in the LAD (left anterior descending coronary artery) with an IMA (internal mammary artery) bypass. Stenoses of the CX (circumflex artery) and/or the RCA (right coronary artery) would, however, be treated with single venous bypasses. In order to ensure a double blind investigation, the patients were separated into two groups (a growth factor group and a control group), each consisting of 20 participants (Figure 15). The conduct of the operation was, as far as the cardiac surgical technique was concerned, identical for both groups. In patients from the growth factor group, however, growth factor plus heparin (0.01 mg FGF-1 per kg body-weight) was introduced immediately after completion of the distal anastomosis, with the extracorporeal circulation (heart-lung machine) still carrying the circulatory burden (Figure 16). Beginning at the level of the IMA-to-LAD anastomosis and continuously infiltrating the myocardium close to the vessel, a solution of physiological saline containing the growth factor was injected alongside the LAD as far as the lower end of the distal stenosis. In the control group, physiological saline alone was used.

In addition to the routine daily laboratory control, the ESR (erythrocyte sedimentation rate) and CRP (C-reactive protein) were determined for all patients of both groups on the 1st, 3rd, and 5th postoperative days, and immediately before discharge. Furthermore, before discharge, each patient was given a final echocardiographical examination, complete with an estimation of the ejection fraction (EF) of the left ventricle.

Follow-up, Control, 12 weeks after operation

Twelve weeks after the Operation, every patient was given a follow-up examination. In addition to a thorough clinical examination, with echocardiographic and laboratory control of the course of recovery, a selective demonstration of the IMA bypass by means of transfemoral intraarterial digital subtraction-angiography (DSA) was performed. A radiologist who did not know whether that particular patient had been given FGF-1 or saline solution during the operation (blinded) undertook this angiographic examination. All angiographs were carried out by the same method: Following bolus administration of 20 ml of water-soluble contrast medium (Solutrast 300®) through an angiographic catheter placed in the femoral artery, the angiographic result was recorded in all patients the same amount of time after injection. The total numbers of angiographic images obtained were subjected to further investigation, and evaluated and compared with each other via computer-supported digital analysis of the grey values. Defined regions of interest were selected for the vessels which had been filled with contrast medium, both in myocardium revascularized by surgery alone, and in myocardium which had also received FGF-1. For each region of interest, 100 image points were further selected and digitally evaluated.

All patients have had follow-up examinations throughout the ensuing 3 years, beginning 3 months after the operation and angiogenic therapy, and continuing thereafter at yearly intervals. Thirty-three patients were available for assessment of laboratory tests and echocardiography at 3 years; 2 patients (out of the control group) refused repeated angiographic examination. Three patients out of the study group (2 x cerebral ischemia and sequelae, 1x unknown) and four patients out of the control group (1x cerebral ischemia, 1x recurrent infarction, 2 x unknown) died in the third year after the operation. Due to the design of the primary study (No. 47/93, Ethical Committee of the University of Marburg), no autopsy studies were performed.

Clinical Investigations
Clinical investigations after 3 years included physical examinations and routine chest X-rays. The actual drug medication was noted, and a comparison between the two groups was carried out.

In a blinded manner, a cardiologist estimated the functional class of each patient, according to the Canadian Cardiovascular Society (CCS) score. All special events related to the cardiovascular system (myocardial infarction (MI), percutaneous transluminal coronary angioplasty (PTCA), redo-coronary artery bypass graft (CABG)) during the 3-year period were recorded. Additionally, at the 3-year follow-up, our ophthalmologist (previously blinded from both groups) examined all patients, with a special focus on retinopathy, corneal, or corpus vitreum disease.

Laboratory Tests

Routine laboratory controls (SMA-12) were performed in all patients at yearly intervals. Also, the tumour markers CEA (Cardiac-Embryonic-Antigen), CA 19-9 (Cancer-Antigen, Marker for Intestinal Carcinoma), NSE (Neuron-Specific-Enolase), and CYFRA (Cytoceratin-Fragment) were recorded in all patients at the 3-year follow-up.

Angiography

The angiographic control of the internal mammary artery (IMA) bypasses and the left anterior descending coronary artery (LAD) systems was performed using a technique identical to the 12-week procedure in 31 patients (17 patients out of the study group and 16 patients out of the control group – i.e., bolus administration of 20 ml water soluble contrast medium (Solutrast 300®, Company Bracco Byk Goulden, Konstanz, Germany) with standardized evaluation of the angiographic records via computer-assisted grey value analysis). The defined areas of interest (i.e., regions of FGF-1 application) were digitally calculated by 100 pixels each, and then compared to the results of the 3-month examination for both groups. Furthermore, neither the radiologist performing the angiography nor the physician conducting the grey value analysis of the angiographic records was informed about the patients' affiliation to either (or both) of the groups.

Echocardiography

Transthoracal echocardiographic was performed in each patient by an independent cardiologist who was blinded with regard to the precise nature of the patients' treatment. In addition to the estimation of the global left ventricular function, the regional wall motion of the anterior wall of the left ventricle was recorded in three segments (basis, mid-portion, and apex).

Statistical Analysis

The results of the first study repeated themselves when all data of the grey value analysis were reported as mean ± standard error of mean (SEM). Comparisons between paired variables were made via students' t-tests. Significance was taken as $P < 0.005$. With regard to the limited number of patients, the echocardiographic data and clinical findings were reported as simple numerical figures.

THE WALL STREET JOURNAL.

© 1998 Dow Jones & Company, Inc. All Rights Reserved.

MEDICINE

Discovery Spurs Heart to Grow Blood Vessels

By RON WINSLOW
Staff Reporter of THE WALL STREET JOURNAL

In a significant advance for the treatment of heart disease, German researchers successfully used genetic engineering to grow new vessels around clogged coronary arteries.

Heart experts said the accomplishment represents an important milestone in an international effort to replace or at least complement coronary-bypass surgery, a widely used treatment for blocked arteries, which are the major cause of heart attacks.

In the first controlled study of the new method, doctors spurred the growth of new blood-carrying vessels in patients' hearts by injecting the patients' heart muscles with a genetically engineered version of a substance the body uses to grow vessels naturally.

The new study is expected to give a boost to several research collaborations between academic scientists and startup companies that are racing to develop techniques to stimulate the growth of new blood vessels. If larger and longer trials are equally successful, doctors believe they will be close to *creating a major new medical procedure easily worth hundreds of millions of dollars a year*.

Researchers at Fulda Medical Center Fulda, Germany, injected a human protein called fibroblast growth factor, or FGF-1, directly into the heart near the obstructed vessels of 20 patients suffering from coronary heart disease. Within four days, a network of tiny new blood vessels sprouted around the diseased arteries of all 20 patients, eventually leading to a new channel that rerouted blood flow around the blockages. Twenty other patients, who were given an inactive form of the growth factor, didn't develop any new vessels.

"With this growth factor we are able to build new vessels," said Thomas-Joseph Stegmann, head of thoracic and cardiovascular surgery at the German facility "That is the important thing we have shown."

Dr. Stegmann heads the research group whose study in today's issue of

Circulation, a journal published by the American Heart Association, is the first published report suggesting that stimulating coronary blood vessel growth through genetic-engineering techniques can work in humans.

"At the moment, we have to say that this procedure isn't replacing bypass surgery," said Dr. Stegmann. "But it could be an additional procedure for vessels that can't be bypassed in the conventional manner.

That alone would be a significant advance for patients, said Stephen Ellis, director of the cardiac-catheterization laboratory at the Cleveland Clinic. About 800,000 patients world-wide undergo bypass surgery each year. Another 800,000 have a less invasive procedure called balloon angioplasty.

"But another 150,000 have severe [chest pain] and aren't candidates for either" procedure, Dr. Ellis said.

"It's an important piece of the puzzle," said Elizabeth Nabel, a gene-therapy researcher and the chief of cardiology at the University of Michigan, Ann Arbor. She noted that several research groups have similar studies under way, most of them focused either on one of several varieties of fibroblast growth factor or on another family of such proteins called vascular endothelial growth factor, or VEGF.

For instance, Genentech Inc., South San Francisco, Calif., is conducting a human trial in which it is injecting bioengineered versions of the VEGF protein into heart patients with the hope of inducing blood vessel growth. **Human Genome Sciences Inc.**, Rockville. Md., is working with Jeff Isner, a gene-therapy researcher at Tufts University School of Medicine, Boston, to develop a therapy that will cause the body's cells to produce VEGF to spur vessel growth. Ronald Crystal, a researcher at New York Hospital **Cornell Medical Center** and founder of GenVec Inc., RockvWe. Md.. began a human trial last month using a VEGF-producing gene. In addition Collateral Therapeutics. San Diego, filed an application to begin a gene-based treatment involving a version

of fibroblast growth factor. It is backed in the venture by Schering AG of Germany.

Dr. Stegmann said his group isn't currently backed by corporate financing. His approach, like the technique Genentech is using with VEGF, isn't gene therapy because it doesn't involve injecting the genes that make the growth factors into the patient where it then works in the cells to produce growth factor proteins. Instead, Dr. Stegmann's group uses biotechnology techniques to produce the growth factor outside the body and then injects the substance directly into the heart. The German group injected the proteins during bypass surgery, but it is expected such, proteins could be administered in the future without open-heart surgery, researchers said. '

All of the patients in the study underwent traditional double or triple bypass surgery to reroute blood flow around blockages in major arteries, but they also had obstructions in other vessels that couldn't be reached easily with bypass, Dr. Stegmann explained. It was at those sites that the researchers injected the protein.

After 12 weeks, images taken of the heart showed substantial growth of new vessels in patients given the treatment and the new network of vessels was seen sprouting from a section of artery above the blockage and rejoining the artery below it, thus circumventing the obstruction, he said.

FIGURE 17: The Wall Street Journal. Article from February 28, 1998, written by Ron Winslow.

11: 2nd Human Clinical Trial (1998-1999)

Having published the results from the first worldwide clinical trial using Angiogenesis as treatment for Coronary Heart Disease *(Circulation 97: 645-650 (1998)* – see Chapter 13), I had it "black on white" that FGF-1 was in fact as effective as I had known all along. FGF-1 really did help grow "brand new" arteries, a network of new vessels. The results of the first clinical trial were not just important to millions of patients throughout the world – it also came as no small surprise to me that the *Wall Street Journal* (Figure 17) wanted to interview me and run an article on my research and the first clinical results. Naturally (although it came as a surprise to me, being a German physician), in strict accordance with the standards of that highly scientific publication, the monetary side of our findings was mentioned. Once FGF-1 was manufactured commercially and the number of patients treated ran into the hundreds of thousands – well, millions, really – the return on an investment in the manufacturing Company (which had yet to be founded) would be enormous.

At about that time, in 1998, *Mr. Dan Montano* entered the picture. Dan Montano was a regular reader of the *Wall Street Journal.* He had sold his Company – a brokerage firm in California – and was looking to invest money and build up a new Company. In addition, *he needed a challenge.* Dan Montano was electrified by what he read about our research and clinical findings. He instantly visualized what this could mean to CHD patients. Dan could serve as my business manager, helping me to recoup something for the effort spent on my research and, naturally, earn more as a reward for my hard work and long-running perseverance.

Dan Montano had been interested in medical topics and news for many years, and he was *a man of action*. He telephoned me right away and told me he would be in Germany the next day to talk with me. I was very surprised but looked forward to meeting this Californian, whose voice and manner I liked from the start. To feel a liking for a person whom I had never met was rather unusual for someone with my emotional makeup; I was more on the reticent side.

When both of us met the next day, we immediately struck the right chord; it was both the start of a reliable, lasting, and deep friendship, and the beginning of the Company later called *CardioVascular BioTherapeutics, Inc.* (CVBT), founded in 1998.

The second human clinical trial was to follow. Before starting, it was important to find ways of producing FGF-1 which were less time-consuming – but where, how? Luckily, Dan Montano, who had been an advisor on foreign affairs to President Ronald Reagan, had good connections to Eastern European countries. One of his main goals had

Patient Data (#20)		
Age		50-77 yrs.
Previous CABG		#13
Previous PTCA / Stent		#6
Target Vessel:	LAD	10
	Cx	3
	RCA	2
	LAD + Cx	3
	LAD + RCA	2

FIGURE 18: Second human clinical trial, Germany 1998–1999. Patient data.

been to bring about a wider opening of the Iron Curtain, and to publicize the principles of capitalism in a positive way. Dan was cognizant of the fact that a team of molecular biologists at the University of Kiev/Ukraine had developed a new process for the manufacture of proteins. Dan and I arranged for a thorough testing of the Ukrainian process in the USA. When the testing was over, there were smiles all around, and I for one was especially relieved: There was indeed a way to produce human proteins – namely FGF-1 – with a dramatically reduced expenditure of money and time. This would greatly stimulate the process of getting FGF-1 to more patients – the number of patients I and other physicians would be able to treat would increase in accordance with the decrease in production expenditure!

The Ukrainian process was patented (*"Phage Process"*), a Sister-Company was founded (*Phage Biotechnology Corporation, Irvine, CA*), and further testing and clinical research would start, replete with new vigour. Thus, Dan Montano's connections to the Ukraine, along with the results of the Kiev University's research, served as a bridge between East and West, one that has since been proven strong and durable.

The first clinical trial was carried out on patients receiving a combination of bypass operation (CABG) *and* FGF-1 injection. It was of the utmost importance that we obtain findings which made clear that the FGF-1 treatment boasted strong efficacy in patients with Coronary Heart Disease. Now, in the second clinical trial, patients would receive the FGF-1 injection as *sole treatment.* These were *no-option heart patients* whose small and calcified vessels were to be treated neither with PTCA nor with surgical revascularization (Figure 18). FGF-1 was their last resort.

Operative Procedure and FGF-1 Administration

Following induction of general anaesthesia, the left hemi-thorax was opened by a limited anterior thoracotomy in the fifth intercostal space. After onset of single lung ventilation, the pericardium was incised in a longitudinal direction. With respect to the three main coronary arteries and their feeding territories (left anterior descending artery (LAD), circumflex artery (CX), right coronary artery (RCA)), and according to the preoperative SPECT findings, the target regions (i.e., regions of reversible ischemia) of the myocardium were identified. FGF-1 was injected (26 G syringe) into the myocardium with a dose per single injection of 0.01 mg/kg body weight combined with 5.0 units heparin (total volume of the injective: 1.5 ml). 0.5 ml fibrin glue (Tissucol™) was then applied immediately to prevent FGF-1 leakage from the injection site. According to the study protocol, a maximum of three injections per patient was allowed. Following treatment, the pericardial incision was closed by three to four single absorbable sutures. After insertion of a routine chest drain, the thoracotomy was closed in the usual manner. The patients were extubated in the operating room, and then transferred to the cardiac intermediate care unit for 24 hours of routine monitoring. All patients were discharged from the hospital between 3 and 5 days after their operations.

Follow-up

During the immediate postoperative course, the patients were submitted to routinely used hemodynamic monitoring, including ECG, echocardiography, chest X-rays, and routing laboratory parameters. Cardiac isoenzymes and complete blood count were measured daily between postoperative days 1 and 5, and the chest tube was removed on the first postoperative day.

According to the study protocol, all patients underwent re-evaluation at day 45 (±3) and day 90 (±3) following FGF1-140 treatment. Mirroring preoperative procedures, all patients underwent SPECT imaging at rest and stress, coronary angiography, echocardiography, ECG, chest X-ray, and exercise testing. Also, serum chemistry, complete blood count, and coagulation parameters were evaluated. Additionally, the following tumour-markers were measured at days 45 and 90, and compared to the preoperative values: Carcino-embryonic antigen (CEA), Carbohydrate antigen (CA 19-9), Cytokeratin fragment (CYFRA 21-1), Alpha Fetoprotein (AFP), neuronal-specific Enolase (NSE), and Prostate-specific antigen (PSA). An experienced ophtalomolgist performed eye examinations with special emphasis on alterations of the retina and corpus vitreum.

SPECT Myocardial Perfusion Imaging

Standardized serial SPECT imaging using ^{99m}Tc-sestamibi in all patients was performed during preoperative rest and stress, and while following up (days 45 and 90, respectively). 2250 MBq ^{99m}Tc-sestamibi were used for studying patients at rest; 750 Mb1 for the stress examination (exercise stress test). All patient studies were acquired via a Siemens SPECT gamma camera; a conventional algorithm was applied for 3-D data reconstruction and display. Performance of myocardial perfusion at rest and stress was evaluated on short axis, vertical axis, and sagittal long axis slices, resulting in a set of 36 slices per investigation. Regarding the region of interest (i.e., the myocardium that had received the FGF-1 injection), a set of 4 short axis slices provided the basis for further evaluation by two blinded observers, using a visual semi-quantitative score. This ranged from 0 (= no perfusion) to 4 (= normal perfusion), modifying the technique according to Berman et al.[15] These scores were added to yield a summed rest score (SRS) and a summed stress score (SSS).

Exercise Protocol

The maximum working capacity of every individual patient was assessed via standardized preoperative bicycle exercise testing (baseline), and at days 45 and 90, too. Strain was increased in 25-Watt intervals every two minutes. The maximum working capacity was determined to be that level of workload which is obtained before the occurrence of either significant changes of ST-segments (>0.2 mV) or angina symptoms.

Statistical Analysis

All data are expressed as mean $\pm$ SD. Continuous variables were compared using paired students' t-tests (baseline and follow-up). A p-value lower than 0.05 was considered to be statistically significant.

12: FDA-guided US Human Clinical Trial (2003)

Based on the previous results in Germany, in March 2002 the FDA approved of and monitored a groundbreaking US Clinical Trial: "Cardio Vascu-Grow™ for the treatment of Coronary Heart Disease." The first US patient treatment using FGF-1 occurred on November 5, 2003, at the University of Cincinnati Medical Center. It was a phase I/II, open label, dose-escalating study to evaluate the safety, tolerability, pharmacokinetics, and effectiveness of human Fibroblast Growth Factor-1 (FGF-1) administered via intramyocardial injection for the treatment of Coronary Heart Disease.

The design of the clinical trial followed that of the second German trial – treating patients with end-stage Coronary Heart Disease with no option of either interventional (PTCA) or operative (CABG) procedures. The inclusion criteria were chronic stable angina refractory to medical treatment, diffuse one-/two-/three-vessel disease, LV ejection fraction greater than 30 percent, age below 25 years, proof of ischemic myocardium while at rest and/or under stress, and a unanimous vote by the Cardiologist and the Cardiovascular Surgeon in favour of the angiogenic treatment. Exclusion criteria were CABG, PTCA, or TMR within 6 months previously, cancer, infection, concomitant heart disease (such as valve disease), renal insufficiency requiring dialysis, and pregnancy.

There were three dosage groups*:
1) 1µg/kg (total dose: 2 µg FGF-1/kg)
2) 3 µg/kg (total dose: 6 µg FGF-1/kg)
3) 10 µg/kg (total dose: 20 µg FGF-1/kg)
   *12 patients per dosage group.

As of this writing (December 2004) 12 patients have been treated (lowest dosage group) without any serious side effects, and with remarkable improvement in the absence/decrease of angina. Improved working capacities have been observed across the board, and some of the patients are now back to working full-time.

The US Clinical entities involved in that trial are:

- University of Cincinnati Medical Center, Cincinnati, OH
- Penn State University Medical Center, Hershey, PA
- St. Joseph's Hospital, Towson, MD
- St. Vincent's Hospital, Bridgeport, CT
- JFK Hospital, West Palm Beach, FL
- University of Alabama Medical Center, Birmingham, AL

A post-treatment interview of the first three US patients was aired nationwide from ABC Headquarters in New York. I presented each of the three patients with a bouquet of flowers. There were smiles all around, and the first patient ever treated in the US, a middle-aged woman, had tears in her eyes. She was so grateful that the horrible pain in her chest had vanished after the treatment, and that she was able to return to her job.

The male patient said it was a miracle. He felt that within a couple of weeks after the treatment with FGF-1, his blood supply experienced a boost.

ABC put the workings of FGF-1 into simple words that could be understood by everyone watching that interview: *"Due to this protein growth factor, brand new arteries are grown from scratch."*

Yes, this outcome made it all worthwhile – the long years of research, laboratory work, and endless nights. FGF-1 actually gave patients a new lease on life, reduced or totally eradicated their chest pain, and helped them get back to work. They did not just survive – *they lived!*

Section IV: Results of Angiogenic Treatment in Humans

13: New Blood Vessels

Results: 1st Clinical Trial

We were able to obtain the human growth factor FGF-1 from each of 40 bacterial cultures of *E. coli*, after separation, purification, and characterization. Upon attaining qualitative proof of the presence of the factor and ensuring its complete purification with HPLC, we had collected 1 mg (± 0.2 mg) of lyophilized FGF from each culture.

The random separation of the 40 patients in the two groups yielded a growth factor group with an average age of 58.1 years (± 6.9 years) and a control group with an average age of 57.8 years (±7.2 years). The former group contained 14 men and 6 women; the latter group, 12 men and 8 women. The preoperative ejection fraction of the left ventricle amounted to 50.3 percent in the growth factor group and 51.5 percent among the controls. These values were satisfactorily comparable. In all 40 patients, we were able to establish the planned bridging over of the proximal LAD stenosis with an internal mammary bypass. In the growth factor group, there was an average of 2.7 single-vein bypasses in the CX or RCA systems, with the corresponding figure for the controls at 2.9. In neither group was a sequential venous or IMA bypass established.

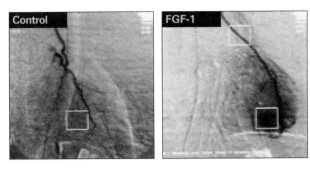

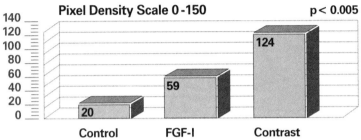

FIGURE 19: First human clinical trial: Proof of neoangiogenesis by grey value analysis of coronary angiograms. Threefold increase of vessel density in the FGF-1-treated patient group.

In no patient taking part in this study did a relevant myocardial ischemia or infarct appear between the time of the operation and the time of discharge from the ward. No significant difference between the two groups was revealed by either the routine daily follow-up examinations or the additional determination of the ESR and CRP carried out on the 1st, 3rd, and 5th postoperative days and immediately before discharge. The patients spent an average of 6.7 days in the hospital after the operation. The final echocardiographic examination of every patient before discharge showed no significant improvement in the average ejection fraction of the left ventricle, compared with the preoperative value, in either group. This is what we had anticipated. The presence of an appreciable (i.e., more than 200 ml estimated by echocardiography) quantity of fluid in the pericardial space could definitely be excluded in both groups.

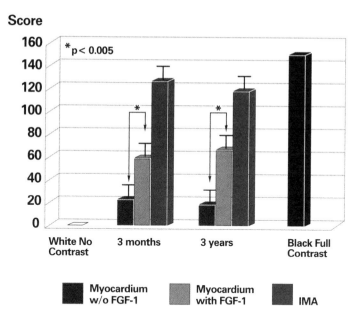

FIGURE 20: First human clinical trial: Persistence of the angiogenic result throughout three years.

It was possible to carry out follow-up examinations on all 40 patients from the two groups 12 weeks after the operation. In each case, we succeeded in obtaining a selective demonstration of the IMA/LAD bypass and the outflow region of the LAD by passing an angiographic catheter through the right femoral artery. As a result of the first clinical use of the human growth factor FGF-1 on the human heart, we were able to produce the same impressive *"in vivo angiogenesis,"* with angiographic confirmation of the new vascular structure that we had already observed during our previous experiments on rats and rabbits.

The angiographs of all 20 patients in the growth factor group showed a decisive difference in comparison with those of the controls. A significant enrichment of contrast medium uptake was recognized clearly in each case where growth factor had been deposited around the LAD (Figure 19). This area of enrichment went beyond the peripheral stenosis of this vessel (or of its side branch), reaching as far as the end of the artery.

The capillary net sprouting from the original coronary artery was able to revascularize the main vessel beyond the subsidiary distal stenosis, a result that could not be achieved via surgery. A similar enrichment of the deposition of the medium around the LAD was not recorded in any patient from the control group, although in all cases the IMA-to-LAD anastomosis could be shown to provide a regular flow of the contrast medium into the LAD. Furthermore, comparing the pre- and postoperative angiographs most definitely excluded the development of new stenoses.

When evaluating the angiography via digital computer-supported analysis of the grey values, a complete blackening of the film was taken as equivalent to a grey value of 150, and an entire absence of blackening to a value of nought. Comparison of the measuring surfaces showed the medium-filled *coronary vessels* to have a value of 124, and those of the surgically treated *myocardium* (without FGF-1), a value of 20. Evaluation of the FGF-1-treated *myocardium* revealed a value of 59, which corresponds to a roughly threefold increase of the value found in the control groups (Figure 19).

FGF-1 really did initiate the growth of brand new arteries – a network of new vessels! We published these findings in *Circulation (Circulation 97: 645-650 (1998))*. I was deeply touched that *J. Folkman*, the *"father of angiogenesis,"* whose previous research and articles were the "firing pin" which set my train of thoughts off in the direction I was soon to take, lauded my research and called this a *"landmark paper."* Now I was slowly

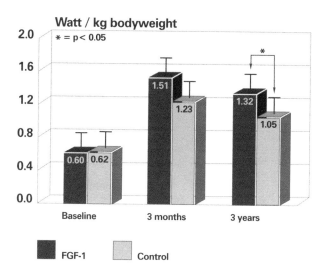

FIGURE 21: First human clinical trial: Improvement of patients' working capacity even three years after FGF-1 treatment.

realizing that my thoughts and dreams had become true – my journey had not yet reached its destination, but I was getting closer. More clinical trials were to follow, but the greatest difficulties had been solved; most obstacles had been cleared.

1st Clinical Trial: Three-Years Results

During the 3-year follow-up period, no patient required redo bypass surgery, and one patient (out of the control group) needed PTCA for stenosis of the circumflex artery (CX), the venous graft to the CX being occluded. All IMA bypasses remained patent with two mild (< 50 percent) stenoses at the IMA-to-LAD anastomosis (one per each group); until now, neither required additional procedures or PTCA. All patients were on continuous medical treatment with Aspirin (100 mg/d) following the operation. One patient, each out of the FGF-1 group, needed nitrate (N), resp. calcium channel blocker (CCB) medication (6 percent vs. 56 percent (N)), and 6 percent vs. 63 percent (CCB) in the control group).

Also, the medication with beta blocker (BB) and ACE-inhibitors (ACE) was diminished in the FGF-1 group as compared with the controls. Related to these findings, the affiliation of the patients to their functional class of CCS was different 3 years after treatment for both groups: 94 percent of the FGF-1 patients were in Class I and 6 percent in Class II, compared with 75 percent of the control patients being in Class I and 25 percent in Class II.

As I've explained, the 3-month angiographic findings for all 20 patients in the study group are completely different from those in the control group. The perivascular area of the LAD, where FGF-1 had been injected – either aimed toward an occluded/stenotic diagonal branch or a distally occluded LAD – showed a significant increase in contrast medium deposit as compared to the controls. These findings were identically evident in the 3-year controls (Figure 20, Figure 21), particularly when visualizing occluded diagonal branches or the distal LAD, depending on the original pathology (Figure 22, Figure 23). Furthermore, there was no recognizable progress or further increase of the neo-vascularization to indicate an uncontrolled vascular growth within the course of 3 years. Comparing the values of the grey value analysis for the FGF-1-group to those of the control group, we found a significant ($P < 0.005$) difference in the 3-month scores: 59 (FGF-1 group) and 20 (control group), respectively. This difference was nearly the same after 3 years: 65 for the myocardium treated by FGF-1; 18 for the controls ($P < 0.005$). However, no significant change in the grey value analysis score was found for the contrast medium filling the IMA and the LAD: 124 after 3 months, and 118 after 3 years. The determination of the general left ventricular ejection fraction (EF) by echocardiography throughout the follow-up period showed a trend toward a better myocardial function for the FGF-1-treated patients' group. From an average of 50.3 percent

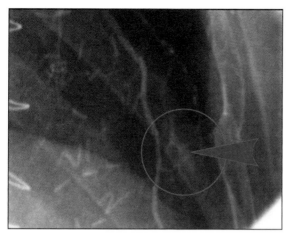

FIGURE 22:
Coronary angiogram of a patient treated by FGF-1 in the diagonal branch area: Three months' result.

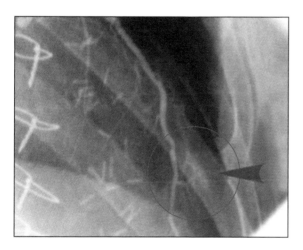

FIGURE 23:
Coronary angiogram of the same patient as in Figure 22: Persistent improvement of myocardial perfusion after three years.

INSERT: Three-year anniversary of the patients.

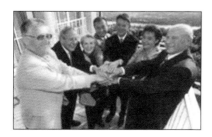

prior to operation and FGF-1-injection, the EF increased to 63.8 percent after 3 years; whereas the EF of the control group went up from 51.5 percent preoperatively to 59.4 percent 3 years after the operation. Looking at the regional function of the three segments of the left ventricular anterior wall, we found, especially for the apical region, a better function in the FGF-1 group: 16 patients had a normokinetic apex, compared to nine patients from the control group. Summarizing the echocardiographic results of the regional left anterior wall motion, there was a higher score (+18.75 percent) for the control group than for the FGF-1 group (+1.96 percent), indicating echocardiographically superior functioning of the left ventricular (LV) anterior wall in the FGF-1-treated patients' group.

Regarding the laboratory findings, there was basically no difference between the groups – especially since the values for the different tumour markers were all in the normal ranges, as in the routine chest X-rays where no abnormalities were found. Repeated examination of the patients' eyes also gave no indication of neo-vascularization of the retina, corpus vitreum, or cornea.

14: Functional Improvements – Results of the 2nd Clinical Trial

Nineteen male patients aged between 50 and 77 years (mean: 63.4 ± 7.17) and one 62-year-old woman were included in this study. All had had advanced and/or diffuse coronary artery disease not amenable for PTCA and CABG (as voted on independently by the cardiologist and cardiac surgeon). Prior to FGF-1 treatment, one patient was in Class II according to the Canadian Cardiovascular Society (CCS), 16 patients were in Class III, and three patients were in Class IV. Previous CABG procedures were performed in 13 patients (twice in two of them), and PTCA in 6 patients. There were seven diabetic patients, three of which were insulin-dependent, and one patient had received an AICD device two years previously due to recurrent ventricular fibrillation episodes. Assessed by echocardiography and ventriculography, the left ventricular EF at baseline ranged from 40 to 85 percent (mean: 64.4 ± 13.39). At baseline stress test, the maximal working capacity ranged from 50 to 150 watts (mean: 96.25 ± 26.54). According to the baseline nuclear perfusion images prior to FGF-1 treatment, the areas of transient myocardial ischemia were identified as follows: LAD supplied area in 10 patients, CX in three, and RCA in two. Three patients showed ischemia in both the LAD and CX regions, and two patients in both the LAC and RCA regions – thus resulting in a total of 25 FGF-1 injections in 20 patients.

There were no deaths or major complications throughout the course of the study. The operations lasted from 42 to 71 minutes (mean: 55.85 ± 9.09). The heart rate and mean arterial blood pressure remained basically unchanged during both the operative and postoperative periods. Blood loss during the operations was minimal; no patient required a blood

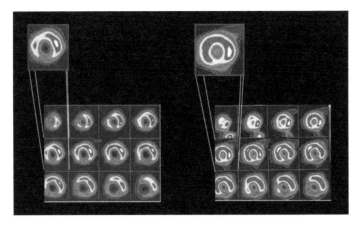

FIGURE 24: Second human clinical trial. SPECT perfusion images at rest. FGF-1 treatment in the LAD-area.

transfusion. In one patient, atrial fibrillation occurred intraoperatively, with spontaneous recurrence of a regular sinus rhythm within 12 hours postoperatively. The postoperative ECGs and the course of the values for the cardiac isoenzymes remained unchanged and showed no evidence of myocardial ischemia in any of the patients.

In all patients, the chest drain could be removed within 24 hours postoperatively. In one patient a left pleural puncture was necessary on day 21 to remove 800 ml of sterile pleural effusion. Another patient suffered from a mild pericardial effusion on day 3, but did not require invasive treatment.

Serial echocardiography throughout the study course failed to show a statistically significant improvement of left ventricular function (EF): 64.4 percent $\pm$ 13.73 (baseline), 65.95 $\pm$ 11.37 (day 45), 64.20 $\pm$ 14.81 (day 90) (p = NS). Capillary density improvement in the area of FGF-1 injection was noted via repeated standardized coronary angiography in all patients, but not evaluated quantitatively. However, no progress of

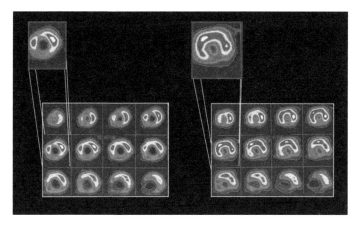

FIGURE 25: Second human clinical trial. SPECT perfusion images at stress. FGF-1 treatment in the LAD-area.

coronary artery disease or plaque-progression in the native coronary vessels or bypass grafts was to be found.

Regarding the clinical status (CCS score): At day 90, 18 patients (90 percent) showed an improvement of at least one class; in four patients an improvement of *two* classes was demonstrated; in two patients the clinical status remained the same as it was preoperatively (Figure 29, Figure 31).

SPECT Myocardial Perfusion Imaging

A total of 120 sets of serial SPECT imaging slices, with 12 slices per investigation, were evaluated (Figure 24, Figure 25). In direct, blinded comparison, the treated myocardial areas (i.e., FGF-1 injection) were scored from 0 (= no perfusion) to 4 (= normal perfusion), comparing the baseline, 45 days, and 90 days images (Figure 30).

Regarding to the SPECT Images series taken at rest, in correspondence to the preoperative (baseline) images, no significant changes could be detected during the course of the study: The summed rest score (SRS) for

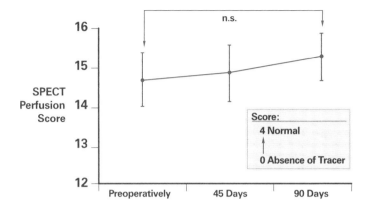

FIGURE 26: Second human clinical trial. SPECT perfusion score at rest.

the areas of interest ranged from 14.70 (±1.34) at baseline to 14.90 (±1.21) at day 45, and to 15.25 (±0.91) at day 90 (p = NS). These findings excluded any adverse effect on the myocardial perfusion due to FGF-1 injection. In contrast to the SRS, the summed stress score (SSS) demonstrated a clear and significant improvement of myocardial perfusion within the treated area: 5.15 ± 2.03 (baseline), 9.70 ± 2.05 (day 45), 10.75 ± 2.21 (day 90) (p < 0.001). Following FGF-1 injection, 21 out of 25 treated areas (84 percent), or 16 out of 20 patients (80 percent), showed a significant increase in tracer uptake during stress SPECT imaging throughout the study period – thus substantiating the increasing values of SSS in the study population (Figure 26, Figure 27).

Working Capacity

Maximal working capacity increased in 16 out of the 20 patients (80 percent) following FGF-1 treatment. From the initial, preoperative mean working capacity of 96.25 (± 26.54) Watts, the study group experienced

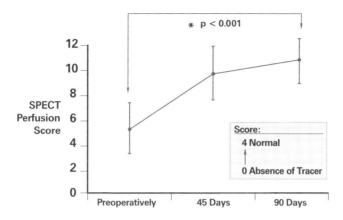

FIGURE 27: Second human clinical trial. SPECT perfusion score at stress.

an increase of maximal working capacity up to 113.75 (± 32.69) Watts at day 45 (p = NS), and then increased up to 123.35 (± 32.50) Watts at day 90 (p < 0.001). Four patients stayed at their pre-treatment levels of maximal working capacity; however, a deterioration of working capacity did not occur in any of the patients (Figure 28).

In 1999, I received an invitation from the Annual Congress of the American Heart Association to present the data from our first human trial. The American Heart Association had issued the following statement: *"Induction of angiogenesis for treatment of coronary heart disease is the number one research advance in 1998."* I considered this to be quite an honour, an astounding acknowledgment of my work. I was greatly looking forward to sharing my experience with other specialists in my field.

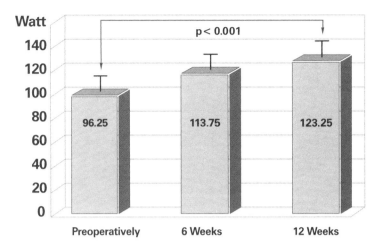

FIGURE 28: Second human clinical trial. Increase of working capacity after FGF-1 therapy.

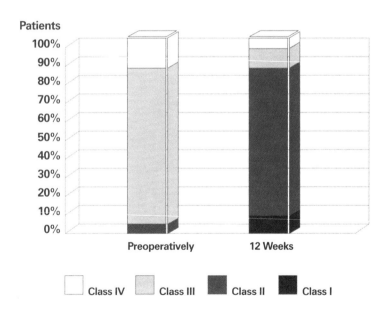

FIGURE 29: Second human clinical trial. Reduction of Angina after FGF-1 treatment.

CCS = CANADIAN CARDIOVASCULAR SOCIETY

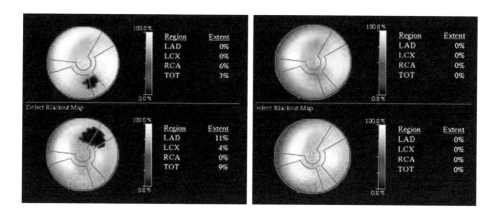

FIGURE 30: US clinical trial (University of Cincinnati, OH). Pre- and postoperative SPECT findings. Normalization of myocardial perfusion after FGF-1 treatment.

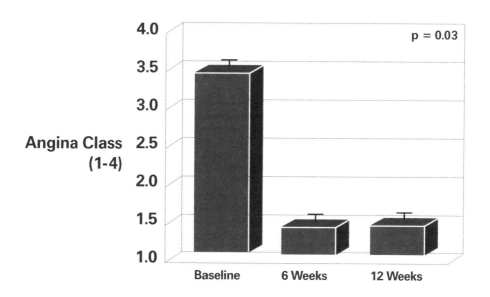

FIGURE 31: US clinical trial (University of Cincinnati, OH). Decrease of Angina score after FGF-1 treatment.

15: Side Effects

Potential Adverse Effects of FGF-1 Delivery

As mentioned above, no deaths or major adverse effects were ascertained during the whole course of study (Figure 23, Figure 33). Focusing on the question of potential oncogenic effects following growth factor therapy, throughout the study we carefully evaluated various tumour markers and their concentration in the serum. Via the use of six different, well-established tumour markers, a wide spectrum of various malignancies was covered: CEA for gastrointestinal tumours; CA 19-9 for pancreatic, gastric, and colorectal cancer; CYFRA 21-1 for all types of lung cancer, particularly the squamous cell carcinoma; AFP for hepatocellular and non-seminomal testicular carcinoma; NSE for tumours of neuroectodermal and neuroendocrinal origin like insulinoma, carcinoid tumour, pheochromocytoma, neuroblastoma, and small cell lung carcinoma; and PSA for cancer of the prostate. Without exception, the levels of all tumour markers stayed in the normal range in all patients throughout the study; no single tumour marker displayed a detectable trend of elevation (Figure 32).

In addition, the serial ophthalmoscopic controls in all patients definitively excluded any change in status of the retina, the cornea, or the corpus vitreum. There was no indication of strengthened (neo-)vascularization in these tissues.

Tumormarker		Preoperatively	6 Weeks	12 Weeks	Normal Value
AFP	(µg/l)	3,79 (± 2.46)	3,53 (± 2.65)	2,89 (± 3.45)	< 15
PSA	(µg/l)	1,69 (± 2.04)	1,68 (± 2.40)	1,27 (± 2.27)	< 4,0
Cyfra	(µg/l)	0,68 (± 0.39)	0,67 (± 0.37)	0,64 (± 0.54)	< 3,3
CA 19-9	(kU/l)	7,46 (± 7.15)	7,65 (± 7.72)	4,57 (± 5.71)	< 37
CEA	(pmol/l)	10,21 (± 4.77)	9,67 (± 4.54)	6,77 (± 6.06)	< 25
NSE	(µg/l)	12,44 (± 9.41)	13.45 (± 12.32)	7,77 (± 6.36)	< 25

FIGURE 32: Second human clinical trial. Exclusion of oncogenic effects of FGF-1 effects by measuring a variety of tumour markers.

AFP = Alpha Fetoprotein

PSA = Prostate-specific Antigen

CYFRA = Cytokeratin fragment

CA 19-9 = Carbohydrate Antigen

CEA = Carcino-embryonic Antigen

NSE = Neuronal-specific Enolase

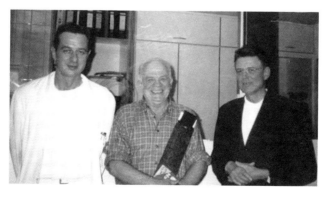

FIGURE 33: Second human clinical trial. A study patient (middle) three weeks after treatment.

> *"He who is not inquisitive*
> *shall not experience anything."*
>
> JOHANN WOLFGANG VON GOETHE, 1749–1832
> GERMAN POET & PHILOSOPHER

Section V: Other Alternatives

Following our publication in *Circulation* (1998), several research groups worldwide were taking up the idea of angiogenesis as a new treatment for Coronary Heart Disease. One of the main approaches used was *gene therapy,* whereby genes encoding growth factors were injected (FGF-1, used by our group, is a (human) protein). Gene therapy using adenovirus mediated gene transfer for encoding VEGF became particularly popular in the field of research and clinical trials.

As it turned out, gene therapy suffered some serious setbacks, so much so that the FDA did not approve human trials in which it was used. In retrospect, I'm grateful to have used the (genetically engineered) growth factor FGF-1 – a *human protein* – and not a gene, especially since the long-term effects after applying protein therapy show no serious side effects.

16: Gene Therapy versus Protein Therapy

Theoretically, angiogenesis can be achieved either by the use of growth factor proteins or by the introduction of genes encoding these proteins. Therapeutic angiogenesis can involve directly administering a vessel growth-promoting substance, such as vascular endothelial growth factor (VEGF) or fibroblast growth factor (FGF). It can also be accomplished using gene therapy – administering genetically engineered viruses, cells, or pieces of DNA that carry the gene encoding VEGF or FGF to patients.

I remember a pivotal discussion about this issue, dubbed "Gene Therapy vs. Protein Therapy," at the 72nd Scientific Sessions of the American Heart Association in Atlanta, Georgia, held between November 7 and 10, 1999. I was invited (and honored) to give a lecture there – entitled *"Therapeutic angiogenesis in the myocardium: Protein delivery"* – and I was the last speaker at the main session. *J. Isner* (Boston) spoke directly before me – favoring gene therapy for the treatment of coronary heart disease. I pointed out my arguments in favor of protein (FGF-1) therapy – mainly the safety advantages of the patients receiving a treatment with a *human protein*, in an *exactly defined dosage*, applied to a *clearly defined area of tissue* (here: the myocardium). After that session I got the impression that the auditorium was mystified by the presumed "elegance" of gene therapy – though it offered little in terms of patient safety. However, later on when serious problems and side effects with gene therapy became apparent, the FDA became very restrictive regarding "gene therapy trials," at which point I thought to myself: *"It was good to remain rational – and to never have forgotten the safety of my patients."*

Therapeutic angiogenesis with VEGF or FGF has been explored for the past 14 years. In 1991, scientists led by *Stephen H. Epstein* of the National

Institutes of Health studied the effects of FGF on the heart vessels of animals. A year later, *Paul Friedman* and his co-workers at Baystate Medical Center in Springfield, Massachusetts, demonstrated that FGF injections could prompt angiogenesis in the hind limbs of rabbits. In the mid-1990s, several groups — including ones led by Epstein, *Michael Simons* of Harvard Medical School, *Jeffrey Isner* of St. Elizabeth's Medical Center in Boston, and *Ronald Crystal* of Cornell University Medical School in New York City — demonstrated that therapy involving angiogenic factors or the genes that encode them could stimulate angiogenesis in the hearts and limbs of animals.

The argument in favor of a gene therapy approach to stimulating therapeutic angiogenesis maintains that gene therapy can overcome the inherent instability of angiogenic proteins by facilitating sustained local production of these angiogenic factors. The arguments against protein therapy follow similar reasoning.

At present, the administration of protein seems to be preferable to gene therapy. This is mainly because dosage modulation in most clinical settings is far easier with purified protein than with gene therapy, which is hampered by the lack of a regulable expression vector. The use of proteins allows the administration of precise amounts of growth factors with a well-defined half-life, pharmacokinetics history, and safety record. Although protein therapy has many advantages, there are, nevertheless, technical problems associated with protein administration, including the optimization of purification and the formulation of delivery for single and/or multiple angiogenic factors.

Recent advances in drug delivery methods using bioerodible polymer matrices will allow for the sustained long-term release of growth factors. This will resolve one of the major problems associated with protein administration: namely, the limited tissue half-life of purified angiogenic factors in patients. An important consideration, however, is that protein therapy be limited to secreted factors. Delivery of intracellular modulators for therapeutic angiogenesis, including transcription factors that control angiogenesis, such as hypoxia inducible factor-1 alpha (HIF-1α), is only possible through gene therapy.

Viral vectors have been the most commonly used means of gene delivery for both VEGF-A and FGF-2. Gene therapy presents an attractive alternative to purified proteins because it offers the potentially sustained production of one or more factors following a single administration. Furthermore, tissue-specific and highly localized production of the therapeutic factor is possible through the use of tissue-specific polymers.

However, a variety of implications warn against the use of viral vectors in gene therapy. Obvious concerns include the potential immune and inflammatory responses to viral vectors. Patients who received VEGF121 via an adenoviral vector had increased levels of serum anti-adenoviral neutralizing antibodies, but there was no report of an inflammatory response in those patients. The use of adenovirus-mediated gene therapy in treating brain tumors has been reported to lead to active brain inflammation as well as persistent transgene expression (up to 3 months after treatment).

The lack of regulable gene expression is another potential barrier. Some systems for inducible gene expressions have proved to be effective and safe amid animal models, but have not yet been tested in humans. Recent advances in stem cell research provide the possibility of combining gene therapy with ex vivo gene transfer into stem cells for angiogenesis therapy. If successful, this approach may overcome most of the obstacles presently presented by gene therapy.

17: Routes of Administration

I deliberated on both the approach of the other research groups and their modes of administering the angiogenic agent. In contrast to the method of application used by these groups – i.e., either intrapericardial, intracoronary, or intravenous infusion/injection – I preferred the administration of FGF-1 to be *intramyocardial*. As it turned out, this was and still is the optimal mode of application, as FGF-1 is administered directly into the diseased target region while those other modes of application distributed the agent into one's overall circulation. That is – to my mind – one of the reasons why the other methods were not convincingly successful.

Intramyocardial Administration

In Germany, I performed one clinical trial (the 2nd Clinical Trial) wherein FGF-1 (Cardio Vascu-Grow™) was administered to no-option heart patients by intramyocardial delivery via a mini-thoracotomy as sole therapy. All patients were discharged from the hospital between postoperative days 3 and 5.

These studies have demonstrated the safety and feasibility of intramyocardial FGF-1 protein delivery as the sole therapy for patients not amenable to percutaneous transluminal coronary angioplasty (PCTA) or coronary artery bypass grafting (CABG). There is persuasive evidence from these trials that intramyocardial FGF-1 application is able to improve myocardial perfusion and maximal working capacity of the treated patients. In the future, intramyocardial application of angiogenic growth factors could emerge as a new treatment – either as an adjunct to bypass surgery or as the sole therapy for patients with advanced coronary artery disease. Other routes of administering an angiogenic agent – such as intrapericardial, intracoronary, or intravenous infusion/injection – were exercised in various trials ... without convincing results.

In addition, the exact same technique was chosen for the actual US clinical trial: intramyocardial injection of FGF-1.

Adjunct to Bypass Surgery

Presently, over 750,000 open-heart bypass operations are performed in the US each year. These procedures are invasive and complex. Often, bypass surgery is focused only on the blockage of larger coronary arteries in the patient's heart; however, smaller vessels may also be experiencing some degree of blockage. In fact, in recent years it has become "normal" for increasingly older patients to suffer from a combination of "proximal" coronary disease and diffuse disease in the periphery of the coronary artery system. In the past, no medical treatment was available for (re-)opening these smaller blocked vessels. CardioVascular BioTherapeutics, Inc. (CVBT) believes that in 70 percent of all open-heart bypass operations, both the patients and their physicians would – given the facts – support injecting Cardio Vascu-Grow™ into those smaller blood vessel sites where blockages exist. The anticipated additional cost of Cardio Vascu-Grow™ as an *adjunct treatment* should be readily acceptable to the vast majority of heart patients and their physicians when compared to the overall cost of open-heart surgical procedures.

Catheter-based Delivery

Patients and cardiologists have something in common: Neither like surgery. Of course, there is a difference between needing a surgical procedure (opening the chest to inject FGF-1 intramyocardially under direct view of the surgeon) and getting a procedure which is very similar to cardiac catheterization. The latter can be done on an ambulant basis: the patient can leave the hospital on the day of the treatment, which is conducted via catheter guided injection of FGF-1 *from the inside of the heart (the left ventricle)*. After discussions with many cardiologists worldwide, I found that the possibility of a catheter guided FGF-1 injection into the myocardium constituted a very logical alternative to surgery.

According to the American Heart Association's (AHA) 2004 update, an estimated 12.9 million Americans have Coronary Heart Disease. This report tells us that 12 percent of those with coronary heart disease receive an open-heart bypass operation (CABG) or a balloon angioplasty (PTCA) procedure. Studies indicate that most, if not all, of the 12.9 million Americans with Coronary Heart Disease also suffer from blockages of smaller coronary vessels, referred to as "diffuse coronary heart disease." The most common treatment for these patients entails addressing their symptoms, which include angina, with medications. Cardio Vascu-Grow™ has the potential to treat not the symptoms, but the root cause of the disease as new vessels grow in the ischemic areas.

Toward that objective, CVBT will design and develop a *catheter-based delivery system* to deliver Cardio Vascu-Grow™ to the desired area of the heart with a much less invasive approach. Most patients with diffuse heart disease refuse to undergo a surgical procedure on their hearts until the situation becomes critical. However, the majority of these patients would most likely submit to a much less invasive procedure wherein Cardio Vascu-Grow™ is delivered to the inside of the heart via a catheter. There is a patient population of up to 3 million people that would gladly seek treatment of their coronary heart disease via a catheter system.

CVBT has initiated studies with a nationally known catheter manufacturing company to perfect catheters that permit the administration of Cardio Vascu-Grow™ to the inside of the heart. Catheter-based delivery would be less invasive, and available to a large population of patients that are not eligible for surgery. The ability to deliver Cardio Vascu-Grow™ via catheter will enable interventional cardiologists to perform the entire medical procedure, eliminating the need for cardiac surgery.

18: Vascular Endothelial Growth Factor (VEGF)

Vascular endothelial growth factor (VEGF) has been used in attempts to stimulate angiogenesis. VEGF-A (commonly referred to as simply VEGF) is the key angiogenic growth factor during embryonic vascular development. In fact, the VEGF-A gene is still the only known gene for which disruption of even one allele results in embryonic lethality. The VEGF-A family of polypeptides consists of a number of biochemically distinct isoforms (up to five in humans) that are generated through alternative mRNA splicing of a single gene. The isoforms are named in accordance with the number of amino acids that comprise the proteins. The human isoforms include VEGF121, VEGF145, VEGF165, VEGF189, and VEG206. They bind to receptors on endothelial cells, resulting in their growth, proliferation, and migration. VEGF can be delivered in two ways: The first is as a gene that encodes this peptide, and the second is as a recombinant protein.

The major advantage of VEGF seems to be its specificity pertaining to endothelial cells, but this may also be a disadvantage if it stimulates the growth of only small, non-muscular arteries that are unable to provide adequate blood flow. All VEGF isoforms are very weak mitogens by themselves. This strongly suggests that the biologic effects of these molecules have a lot more to do with mechanisms other than the direct stimulation of endothelial cell proliferation.

Early studies involving the administration of VEGF-A showed angiographic evidence of new vessel formation, but these vessels did not persist; they regressed within three months. One of the major problems encountered in the use of VEGF-A is that the vessels formed are unstable and leaky. Researchers hypothesize that VEFG-A alone may not be sufficient to form stable, mature vessels that are characterized by the recruitment of the perivascular mural cells, such as pericytes and smooth muscle cells. This process of vessel maturation is called arteriogenesis, and is arguably the ideal way to form stable vessels for therapeutic purposes.

19: Transmyocardial Laser Revascularization (TMR)

Transmyocardial Laser Revascularization (TMR) is a procedure used to relieve severe angina or chest pain in very ill patients who are not candidates for bypass surgery or angioplasty. In this technique, the chest is opened surgically and a handheld laser is used to drill from 20 to 40 microscopic openings into the heart muscle and the left chamber of the heart (the left ventricle), improving blood flow to the heart and relieving heart disease-related chest pain or angina. Bleeding from the laser channels on the outside of the heart stops after the surgeon applies pressure with his finger for a few minutes.

No one really knows why TMR helps reduce the pain of angina, but some physicians think that the procedure helps the growth of tiny new blood vessels (angiogenesis) in the heart muscle wall. These new blood vessels bring more blood to the heart muscle, possibly stimulating the growth of new, healthy vessels that can supply the muscle with more oxygen. Others think that the TMR laser destroys nerve fibers to the heart, diminishing patients' ability to feel their chest pain. Still others think that the extremely ill patients are simply experiencing a placebo effect.

Although TMR is in fact surgery, it is done while the heart is still beating and full of blood. A heart-lung machine is not needed, and surgeons do not cut open chambers of the heart, so TMR is not open-heart surgery. The procedure takes about 2 hours and patients typically have hospital stays of between 4 and 7 days.

In an even newer technique known as Percutaneous Transmyocardial Laser Revascularization (PTMR), the laser is delivered via a catheter which is threaded through the artery until it reaches the heart.

Because PTMR only requires a tiny incision at the site of the artery, both the surgery time and recovery times are shorter.

Compared with surgical TMR, this less invasive form of laser treatment provides similar benefits with fewer side effects. Although PTMR has been proven to be safe and feasible, it is not clear if the treatment is effective. Survival rates have been similar in both groups. A number of patients in both groups end up needing angioplasty, bypass surgery, or other treatment.

Neither TMR nor PTMR will replace coronary artery bypass or angioplasty as the most common method of treating coronary artery disease. These alternatives have simply been proven to be safe, effective ways to restore blood flow to the heart muscle. However, TMR is employed for patients who are high-risk candidates for a second bypass or angioplasty, people whose blockages are too diffuse to be treated with bypass alone, and some patients who develop atherosclerosis after heart transplants.

20: Myogenesis – Stem Cells

Stem cells are cells that have not taken on the identity of any specific cell type and are not yet committed to any dedicated function. They can divide indefinitely and may be induced to give rise to one or more specialized cell types. They not only offer scientists a tool to study the early molecular events in organ development, they also offer hope for tissue repair and regeneration to patients suffering from a wide spectrum of degenerative diseases, including coronary artery disease.

Donald Orlic and colleagues published a paper in *Nature* (2001) suggesting that stem cells derived from bone marrow can replace heart muscle lost as a result of heart attack, thus improving cardiac function. The injection of bone marrow stem cells into an injured heart seemed to constitute a new therapy, triggering the launch of many clinical studies investigating the effect of directly injecting these cells into the damaged heart muscle of heart attack patients.

This initial enthusiasm was put to the test by successive experiments using several types of stem cells, which showed that transdifferentiation occurs rarely, if at all, in many organ systems, including the heart muscle. The observed plasticity of adult stem cells might be explained by simple cell fusion rather than reprogramming. In addition, a recent clinical study in which bone marrow stem cells were transplanted into injured hearts was terminated due to serious cardiac side effects that threatened the blood flow to the heart. Clearly, further experimental testing is necessary in large animal model systems.

In other clinical studies, ones which used patients' own myoblasts (progenitors of non-cardiac muscle cells) in the hope of increasing the amount of viable muscle after a heart attack, it was shown that transplanted myoblasts can improve heart function. Patients' own myoblast cells were directly injected into their injured hearts. Although there were reports of abnormal heartbeats, an overall improvement in heart function was observed.

The chief task is to find the ideal source of cells. Previous results suggest that fetal heart cells might be the optimal cell type for heart-cell transplantation therapy. Embryonic cells are the ancestral cells of every cell in the body. In a developing embryo, they transform into cells that ultimately make up one's organs, bone, skin, and other tissues. Embryonic stem cells can spontaneously transform into vessels and organize themselves in a pattern like that which occurs during the formation of an embryo. Nevertheless, the controversy that surrounds their use in scientific research ensures that they will not be used in clinical studies, at least not for the near future.

Section VI: The Future

I am a cardiovascular surgeon – and that entails the daily experience of performing surgical procedures on the *entire cardiovascular system:* the heart, the aorta, the arteries, the veins. Because of the importance of heart diseases, which are the main cause of death in the Western world (particularly coronary artery disease), my research regarding angiogenesis was initially focused on the heart.

However, atherosclerotic disease is a *systemic disease,* and it is common for cardiovascular surgeons to see patients with coronary heart disease whose entire arterial systems are *also* (more or less) involved in the pathological process of atherosclerosis.

While my friend Dan Montano and I travelled around the world, we talked a lot. Naturally, we talked about the basics of life, about philosophy and history, about the diversity of societies and countries, about women and men and their relationships – however, we also talked about the potential of FGF-1. Dan Montano became my "medical student" – just as I became his "business student." On a trip back from Asia, where we were faced with a disease named *"BUERGER's Disease"* (i.e., atherosclerotic disease of the peripheral arteries of the legs, common among men – and smokers), which is prevalent in Asia and India. And there is no good treatment available for its patients – so amputation is often called for. Also, among diabetics, it is common for atherosclerosis to involve the periphery of the arterial system – with no option for interventional or surgical treatment. *"Why,"* I said to Dan, *"not use the principle of angiogenesis for these patients? It is the same disease – atherosclerosis."*

A new idea was born.

"And what about strokes?" Dan asked me from across the aisle on another flight from Japan to Europe.

"Yes, you are right," I answered. *"And even more important: these patients suffering from strokes as a manifestation of atherosclerosis of the cerebral vessels have nothing to lose."*

Another step into the future had been taken.

We discussed the problem of wound healing – a natural process of human tissue often complicated and disturbed by a lack of arterial perfusion and oxygen supply. Why not use the power of FGF-1 to increase the blood supply to wounds? The first series of experiments with CVBT has already been finished – with astounding results.

Furthermore, as one of the most powerful "steering proteins" in the human body, FGF-1 also has the potential to repair and regenerate neurons and nerve cells. Many neurological disorders, to some extent not fully understood regarding their origins and mechanisms, display the common phenomenon of "degenerating" neurons and nerve fibres: Spinal cord injuries, Peripheral (often: diabetic) Neuropathy, Parkinson's Disease, Amyotrophic Lateral Sclerosis, Multiple Sclerosis ... and there is no sensible treatment available for these diseases. So a new research section of CVBT was built – with the goal of developing a new treatment based on the potency of this powerful protein, FGF-1 (Figure 34).

FGF-1 (CardioVascuGrow™) Medicated Neo-Angiogenesis

Indications (Future, Research)

- Ischemic Cardiomyopathy (Angiogenesis <u>PLUS</u> Myogenesis)

- HTx-Recipients: Transplant Vasculopathy

- Cerebrovascular Disease (FGF-1 → Repair of Neurons) [J. Clin. Invest. 112, 2003: 1202-1210]

- Anastomoses (e.g. Bronchial Tree, Intestinal Tract)

- Wound Healing

- Acute Myocardial Infarction (?)

FIGURE 34: Overview of future indications for FGF-1 treatment.

21: Peripheral Vascular Disease (PVD)

Lower extremity "Peripheral Vascular Disease" (PVD) occurs in the blood vessels (arteries) of the back and legs. PVD is often called "Peripheral Artery Disease" (PAD), or atherosclerosis, and is a progressive disease that involves the calcification and narrowing of the arteries due to a gradual buildup of plaque. PVD of the lower extremities is a major cause of diminished ability to walk, and advanced cases can lead to leg amputation. The primary symptom of lower extremity PVD is a type of leg pain ("claudicatio intermittens") that occurs when a patient is active (e.g., while walking) called intermittent claudication. The pain is caused by inadequate oxygen supply to the legs. In severe cases, patients may experience pain even at rest, and pain due to tissue loss or gangrene. Diabetics are especially at risk of getting PVD.

According to the AHA's 2004 update, PVD affects 8–12 million Americans, and atherosclerotic processes of the lower extremities affect 12–20 percent of Americans aged 65 or older. The mortality per year reaches as high as 122,000 deaths (Figure 35).

The diffuse nature of PVD often makes it difficult to treat. Estimates of PVD's prevalence in the U.S. range from 8-12 million patients, 250,000 of whom are hospitalized annually. Treatment options include angioplasty, stenting, and other catheter-based procedures to dissolve clots. Surgically removing plaque from blood vessels is often necessary to prevent an embolism from forming or to allow for better blood flow through a blocked artery. Bypass grafts are another surgical alternative. In general, surgical procedures carry a higher risk factor and a lower recovery rate, but offer better and longer lasting outcomes.

American Heart Association Report 2004

Peripheral Arterial Disease (PVD)

- 8-12 Million Americans affected
- 12-20% of Americans age 64 and older affected
- Mortality: 122,200 per year

FIGURE 35: Impact of peripheral artery disease in the USA. Data from AHA update 2004.

There is a significant need for better therapies. Very promising research supports growing new blood vessels that may improve the blood supply to the back, legs, and feet to promote wound healing and decrease pain. Cardio Vascu-Grow™ has been demonstrated to stimulate the growth of new blood vessels when injected near a blocked coronary artery, leading to a significant increase of blood flow around the blockage. It is hoped that this success can be duplicated in the back and legs.

Cardio Vascu-Grow™ is in the animal testing phase, and is aimed at diabetics who often suffer from peripheral vascular disease in their backs and legs.

22: Stroke

In 1986, my mother suffered a stroke. Her right internal carotid artery was blocked – giving her son no chance to perform a surgical treatment, such as a carotid endarterectomy. I treated her in the conventional, conservative manner – with no hope of overcoming the sequelae: left-sided hemi paresis, intermittent entanglement, partial memory loss ...

Everybody who has had a stroke victim in his family is familiar with this dire situation. After five years of devoted care and nursing, particularly at the hands of my sister *Mechthild*, my mother died at age 71 due to the consequences of that stroke. Had there been a chance of treatment with FGF-1 ...

Strokes are a force that know no boundaries: *F.D.Roosevelt, W.S.Churchill, J.W.Stalin* – they all died because of strokes (Figure 36).

Strokes resulting in brain damage are most often caused by a lack of blood flow to a specific part of the brain. A stroke results in permanent damage to the brain tissue – and in many cases, a permanently disabled patient.

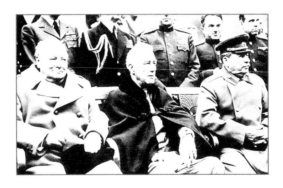

FIGURE 36: Conference of Jalta, Ukraine, February 1945: W. Churchill, Th. Roosevelt, J. Stalin. They all died due to strokes.

American Heart Association Report 2004 (NHLBI):

USA:

700,000 patients per year suffer a STROKE!

280,000 patients per year die because of a STROKE!

FIGURE 37: Frequency of strokes in the USA. Data of the AHA update 2004.

In the United States, strokes are the third leading cause of death and a leading cause of serious, long-term disability. The probability of stroke increases as people get older, with those over age 65 at the greatest risk. According to the American Heart Association (2004), approximately 700,000 Americans suffer a stroke each year; about 40 percent (or approximately 280,000 patients) of whom are killed (Figure 37). On average, someone in the United States has a stroke every 45 seconds. Each year about 40,000 more women than men have strokes. In 2004, the estimated direct and indirect cost of strokes was $53.6 billion.

Even in children, strokes are an issue. Strokes among children peak in the perinatal period: In the National Hospital Discharge Survey from 1980–1998, the rate of strokes among infants less than 30 days old (per 100,000 annual live births) was shown to be 26.4, with rates of 6.7 for hemorrhagic stroke and 17.8 for ischemic stroke.

Ischemic or occlusive strokes, which account for about 88 percent of all strokes, are caused by an obstruction in an artery, generally one of the carotid arteries (and the branches thereof), the major arteries in the neck that carry oxygen-rich blood from the heart to the brain (Figure 38). Only limited treatment is available to patients who have suffered a stroke. Thrombolytic therapy (for example, using rTPA) is sometimes tried in these patients to unblock the arteries supplying blood to the brain, but safety and bleeding issues have prevented this treatment from gaining widespread acceptance in the medical community.

Animal studies have shown the potential of growth factor therapy in limiting the severity of brain ischemia after a stroke. A stroke is characterized by an infracted area of the brain, which is incapable of recovering, surrounded by a minor-perfused area of risk, which would be the target of growth factor treatment. CVBT has initiated animal studies to confirm that Cardio Vascu-Grow™ has the potential to limit brain damage in animals that have experienced an ischemic insult (read: a stroke) to the brain (Figure 39).

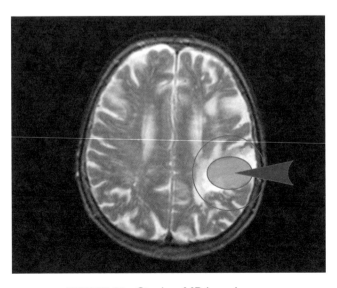

FIGURE 38: Stroke: MR-imaging.

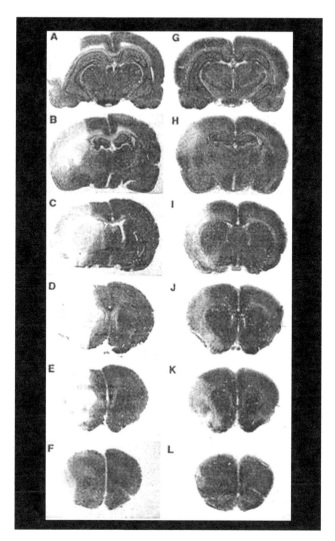

FIGURE 39: Experimental (rats) stroke: Reduction of stroke volume after treatment with FGF-1.

RIGHT: FGF-1 treated animal (brain)
LEFT: Control animal (brain).

23: Anastomoses (Bronchial Tree, Intestinal Tract)

In every type of "resecting" (excising) surgery, there is a need for "reconnecting" the various forms of tissues. This is valid, for example, during surgery for bronchial carcinoma, when a segment or a lobe of the lungs has to be resected due to malignancy. After resection, either a closure of the remaining bronchial tree or a reconnection (anastomosis) has to be performed. Also, after resections of parts of the intestinal tract (say for infections, occlusions, benign tumors, malignant tumors), it is necessary to surgically perform an anastomosis between the remaining parts of the intestinal tract – thus gracing the intestinal pathway with continuity.

It is a general surgical experience (witnessed in numerous animal experiments) that the perfusion, the blood supply, and the oxygenation of such a surgically created anastomosis are *the* critical factors (aside from surgical technique, general condition of the patient, etc.) when it comes to the healing of tissue: the better the blood perfusion of an anastomosis, the lower the risk of leakage. And leakage of an anastomosis, either inside the thorax or inside the abdomen, is always a life-threatening complication which can result in serious infection, sepsis, and even death.

Accordingly, when increasing the local blood supply to any anastomosis, the application of Cardio Vascu-Grow™ could diminish the risk of postoperative leakage and promote the uncomplicated healing of any tissue connections and anastomoses. Research and animal experiments addressing this issue must be performed.

24: Chronic Kidney Disease

According to the 2003 Annual Data Report (ADR) produced by the U.S. government in association with the National Kidney Foundation, approximately 8 million Americans suffer from chronic kidney disease. The senior Medicare population is composed of 5.9 million patients. The incidence and prevalence of kidney disease have doubled in the last 10 years, and are expected to keep growing. This disease damages the circulatory system of the kidney, most often via chronic hypertension. Chronic high blood pressure destroys the small capillaries in the glomerulus, or blood filtering apparatus, of the kidney, leading to permanent kidney damage, kidney failure, and even death.

Americans with chronic kidney disease have high rates of hospitalization for cardiovascular disease. In fact, this population is more likely to see deaths that are cardiac in origin than deaths resulting from end stage renal disease. Antihypertensive drugs are most often prescribed for patients with chronic kidney disease. These include diuretics, beta-adrenergic blockers, calcium channel blocks, and Angiotensin inhibitors.

Animal studies have shown that members of the Fibroblast Growth Factor family, which includes Cardio Vascu-Grow™, can lead to the formation of new blood capillaries in the glomerulus, capable of restoring this organ's blood filtration capacity.

CVBT will initiate animal studies to confirm the efficacy of Cardio Vascu-Grow™ when it comes to stimulating the formation of new blood vessels in damaged kidneys.

25: Wound Healing

Skin Wound Healing

Impaired wound healing is a problem among the elderly, diabetics, and immunosuppressed and immobilized individuals. Impaired healing increases the cost of care as well as the length of time in which care needs to be provided, and it reduces patients' quality of life. Estimates of the cost of treating all chronic wounds run to $5-7 billion per year. This figure is expected to increase by 10 percent annually. An aging population will see an increase in bedridden patients whose fragile skin is resistant to healing. Other estimates state that some 1.5 million of the 14 million diabetics in the United States suffer from impaired healing problems. According to the Health Care Financing Administration (HCFA), the number of lower-extremity, diabetes-related amputations has risen from 56,000 in 1994 to 87,000 in 2000.

The incidence of decubitus, or pressure ulcers (a.k.a. bed sores), is even greater, with 5 million in acute care settings, 1.25 million in long-term health care settings, and 1.1 million in home health care settings. At present, the cost of treating a pressure ulcer can run as high as $50,000, and require several months – or even years – of healing. Given the rate at which the population is aging, this problem will increase dramatically. There is a tremendous need for more effective and affordable wound-healing products. Such products would undoubtedly enjoy strong market acceptance by physicians, patients, and insurers.

An ongoing animal trial has been initiated by CVBT for this indication. Diabetic mice have received surgical wounds and have been treated with differing doses of Cardio Vascu-Grow™. After 60 days, all the mice have healed except for 3/6 of the control group and 1/6 of the highest FGF-1 dosing group (Figure 40).

Corneal Wound Healing

The cornea is the transparent front covering of the eyeball. It is the most sensitive part of the body, and readily reacts to irritants both inside and outside of the eye. Corneal scarring after penetrating injury and/or surgery is a significant cause of visual impairment. A wounded ocular surface may fail to heal properly in a variety of clinical situations, and treatment can be extraordinarily frustrating for even the most knowledgeable cornea and eye expert. A significant number of patients fail to respond to traditional antibiotic treatments. For this reason, "growth factors" which might promote wound healing is currently a topic of substantial interest to the ophthalmology community.

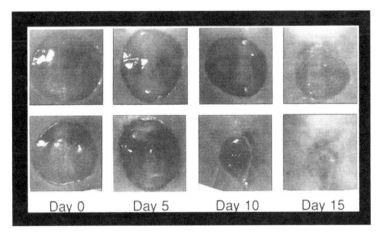

Day 0   Day 5   Day 10   Day 15

FIGURE 40: Wound Healing. Experimental (mice) treatment of wounds by FGF-1.

LOWER LINE: Improved wound healing after FGF-1 application.
UPPER LINE: Control.

The market potential for Cardio Vascu-Grow™ in corneal wound healing is difficult to gauge, but it could be very significant. Eye injuries send 2.4 million people to the emergency room or ophthalmologist each year. A considerable number of these injuries are cornea injuries. About 4 million laser eye surgeries are projected for this year alone. Wound healing and improving surgical outcome constitute an increasingly important market as elective LASIK surgery becomes more and more commonplace. Complications resulting from LASIK occur in approximately 1.5 to 5 percent of all patients.

Veterinarians would make up a large secondary market. Dogs and cats frequently suffer from scratches or abrasions to the cornea (corneal ulcers), making such injuries one of the most common reasons for a visit to the vet. Drugs used by veterinarians for eye injuries (typically antibiotics alone or antibiotics with steroids) are often registered for use in both humans and animals. The human formulations and animal formulations are produced by the same pharmaceutical companies.

26: Neurological Indications

In May 2004, I was in Bridgeport, Connecticut, and had just finished a lecture on angiogenesis for the treatment of coronary heart disease, when a physician from the audience ran up to me, excited and out of breath, and stammered: "Do you think your technique can be applied to the millions of patients in the U.S. who suffer from excruciating lower back pain? I have heard about lumbar ischemia, and perhaps this is caused by blockage of blood vessels to the lower back muscles." I pondered this physician's question and thought perhaps his comment deserved some looking into.

Along with my trusted scientific colleague – and more than that: my friend – *Dr. Jack Jacobs,* a molecular biologist from California and chief scientific officer of our laboratory facility in Irvine, I began to explore whether any research on this topic existed. What we discovered amazed us.

According to a recent article in Forbes magazine, Chronic back pain affects 26 million Americans. It is estimated that up to 8 million of these patients may suffer back pain due to lumbar artery disease, where the blood vessels become blocked by atherosclerotic plaques. We found a series of articles from the University of Helsinki, Finland, by *Leena Kauppila*, M.D., Ph.D., who has championed the idea that a significant percentage of people who suffer from chronic lower back pain have vascular disease in the arteries supplying the muscles and discs of the lower back. She has published extensively on this topic in very prestigious medical journals.

According to Dr. Kauppila, lumbar ischemia occurs when lumbar arteries and their smaller branches are occluded due to a build-up of plaque.

These atherosclerotic lesions decrease blood flow and nutrient supply to the lumbar spine and its surrounding muscle structures, causing disc degeneration and lower back pain. In addition, the ischemic muscle cannot properly remove metabolic waste products that irritate nerve endings in the area, which also contributes to lower back pain. Finally, individuals may adapt to impaired blood flow to their lower back by reducing the amount of physical work they perform. This inactivity can lead to further muscle atrophy and pain, as well as degeneration of the spinal discs in the area (Figure 41).

Treatment options for these patients include pain medications, which only temporarily relieve symptoms and can have serious, even deadly side-effects, and/or back surgery to treat the disc generation, which can sometimes worsen the situation.

Growing new blood vessels that may improve the blood supply to ischemic areas of the lower back is a potential new application for "our" growth factor, FGF-1. As in the heart, where FGF-1 has been demonstrated to stimulate the growth of new blood vessels when injected near a blocked coronary artery, research can now begin with FGF-1 to duplicate this success in the lower back as well. Patients with chronic lower back pain will do anything to relieve themselves of this burden, and FGF-1 may provide them with long-term relief of their debilitating pain.

Spinal Cord Injury

Approximately 250,000-400,000 individuals in the United States have Spinal Cord Injuries (SCI). Every year, approximately 11,000 people sustain new Spinal Cord Injuries. Most of these people are injured in auto and sports accidents, falls, and industrial mishaps.

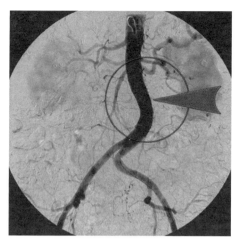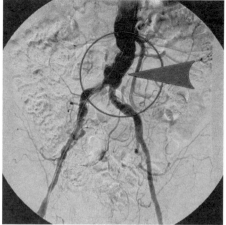

FIGURE 41: Chronic Lumbar Ischemia. Two angiograms of patients suffering from chronic back pain. Angiographies pointed out severe atherosclerotic disease of the distal abdominal aorta – with occluded or stenotic lumbar arteries (arrows).

An estimated 60 percent of these individuals are 30 years old or younger, and the majority of them are men. Severe SCI leads to a devastating loss of neurological function below the level of the injury and adversely affects multiple body systems. By nature, an SCI has a very sudden impact on an individual – physically, emotionally, and socially. One of the most difficult issues to deal with is that there is no "cure" or effective treatment at present.

The spinal cord is an integral part of the body's most specialized system, the central nervous system (CNS). A major role of the spinal cord is to carry messages to and from all parts of the body and the brain through a network of nerves which links the cells of the spinal cord to target cells in all other systems of the body. An individual nerve cell is called a neuron, and each neuron has receptive branching fibers called dendrites. The axon, carrying an output signal, extends from the cell body, and is covered by a protective fatty substance called a myelin sheath, which helps the impulse travel efficiently. Spinal cord injuries sever axons that transmit sensory and motor information. Regenerating these axons and reconnecting them with their target neurons in the brain and spinal cord will lead to improved sensory and motor function in persons with spinal cord injuries.

Currently researched measures attempt to alter the environment around the injury site to encourage nerve cell growth and repair. Peripheral nerves can regenerate due to the presence of cell proteins that stimulate rather than inhibit nerve growth. Nerve "growth factors" that nourish and stimulate the growth of nerve cells have the potential to heal spinal cord injuries. Finding effective ways to introduce these cells or substances into the spinal cord to achieve functional recovery is the major goal of "cure" research today. An investigation of the potential of Cardio-VascuGrow™ to be that cure is most certainly on the agenda.

Peripheral Neuropathy

Peripheral neuropathy is a death of nerve fibers, particularly in the extremities of the feet, legs, and hands. In this disease the protective sheath, or myelin, that protects the nerve degenerates, which results in nerve exposure and subsequent nerve damage. Diabetic Peripheral Neuropathy (DPN) and the associated microvascular (small blood vessel) damage can lead to foot ulcers and amputations. DPN is the leading cause of non-traumatic lower-limb amputations among people with diabetes in the United States. More than 80,000 amputations are performed each year due to DPN. Sensory symptoms of DPN include numbness, prickling, aching pain, burning pain, stabbing pain, and allodynia (a condition in which ordinarily non-painful stimuli, such as a bed sheet touching a leg, invoke pain). Neuropathy can also lead to problems with internal organs. Neuropathy increases in accordance with age, the duration of a case of diabetes, and the worsening of glucose tolerance. Tight blood glucose control is the only way to stop the disease at present, but even that does not always work.

About 17 million Americans have been diagnosed with diabetes, and it is estimated that between 60 and 70 percent of them have some degree of DPN. Approximately 800,000 diabetics in the U.S. are treated annually for symptoms of peripheral neuropathy, with a total annual cost of nearly $11 billion incurred by all payers.

In addition to being a side effect of diabetes, peripheral neuropathy is also a side effect of many anti-HIV therapies, and of HIV itself. About one quarter of all HIV patients will develop sensory neuropathy over a 10-year period. Due to improved drug treatment, HIV patients are living longer, and an estimated 900,000 HIV/AIDS patients live in the United States today. Cancer survivors also experience peripheral neuropathy when they undergo chemotherapy, and are therefore potential candidates for Cardio Vascu-Grow™ treatment.

For symptomatic treatment, doctors often prescribe pain-killing drugs. Pain management tends to be difficult and disappointing, as the drugs do not halt the progression of the neuropathy. The United States currently approves of no prescription therapy designed to target or reverse the underlying process of micro vascular damage that leads to DPN.

Cardio Vascu-Grow™ is presently in the animal testing phase for the treatment of peripheral neuropathy.

Neurological Diseases and Disorders

Given the complexity of neuronal tissue in the human brain, ailments affecting the central nervous system are often difficult to treat. Millions of people suffer from disorders of the central nervous system, and the number is expected to rise as more people live longer. For most of these patients, there are no cures for such diseases. Drug therapies have focused on slowing the progress of the disease. If a drug has shown some effectiveness for one disease, pharmaceutical companies routinely try the same medication "off label" for other neurological diseases, going by the theory that if a drug works on one neurodegenerative disease, it may very well work on other diseases characterized by neuronal loss. Cardio Vascu-Grow™ might well become an effective therapy for several neurological diseases and disorders, beginning with the ones described below ...

Parkinson's Disease

Parkinson's disease is easily one of the most baffling and complex of all neurological disorders. Its cause remains a mystery, but research in this area is active, with new and intriguing findings constantly reported. The signature of the disease is the loss of brain cells that produce a chemical called dopamine, which helps direct muscle activity. The constant shaking and tremors that affect Parkinson's patients greatly interfere with daily activities. The disease is both chronic and progressive, meaning the symptoms steadily worsen over time. About 50,000 Americans are diagnosed with Parkinson's disease each year, and more than half a million Americans are affected at any given time. The average age of onset is 60. According to the National Parkinson Foundation, each patient spends an average of $2,500 a year on medications. After factoring in office visits, Social Security payments, nursing home expenditures, and lost income, the total cost to the U.S. is estimated to exceed $5.6 billion annually. At present there is no cure for Parkinson's disease, but a variety of medications do provide relief from the symptoms. Levodopa (L. dopa) is the gold standard of present Parkinson's drug therapy. Nerve cells can use levodopa to make dopamine and replenish the brain's dwindling supply. It delays the onset of debilitating symptoms, extending the period of time in which patients can lead relatively normal, productive lives.

Unfortunately, levodopa becomes less effective over time, and many patients suffer serious side effects.

Amytrophic Lateral Sclerosis (ALS) – "Lou Gehrig's Disease"

ALS is a progressive neurodegenerative disease that attacks nerve cells in the brain and spinal cord. When motor neurons die, the ability of the brain to initiate and control muscle movement is lost. With all voluntary muscle action affected, patients in the later stages of the disease are totally paralyzed. Yet, through it all, the vast majority of people's minds remain unaffected. About 5,600 people in the U.S. are diagnosed with ALS each year. It is estimated that as many as 30,000 Americans have the disease at any given time. The incidence (number of cases in the population) of ALS is five times greater than that of Huntington's disease and about equal to that of multiple sclerosis. Half of all people affected with ALS live at least three or more years after diagnosis. Twenty percent live five years or more; up to 10 percent will survive for more than 10 years. The financial cost to families including people with ALS is exceedingly high. Estimates state that in the advanced stages, when the patient is functionally quadriplegic, professional care can cost an average of $200,000 a year.

The present treatment of ALS is aimed at symptomatic relief. Rilutek® is the only drug approved at present. An antiglutamate drug, it appears to slow the progress of ALS, prolonging the life of persons with ALS by at least a few months. Current research is focused on other antiglutamate drugs, as well as Insulin-Like Growth Factor-1 (IGF-1), presently in clinical trials, and vascular endothelial growth factor (VEGF), presently at use in mouse models.

Multiple Sclerosis (MS)

Multiple sclerosis is an autoimmune disease wherein the body's own immune system, which normally targets and destroys substances that are foreign to the body (such as bacteria), mistakenly attacks normal tissue. In MS, the immune system attacks the brain and spinal cord, two components of the central nervous system. The disease manifests itself in a variety of symptoms, ranging from an ever-present tingling or numbness in the limbs, to spasticity and paralysis. These debilitating symptoms are caused by the destruction of the protective myelin sheath (demyelination) surrounding nerves in the central nervous system. This demyelination disrupts the normal transmission of electrical impulses along the nerves of the brain and spinal cord. The most common form of MS is relapsing-remitting, in which patients cycle into relapses that beget almost total recovery. In contrast, secondary progressive MS is less common but more severe, with a gradual progression of disability following an initial cycle of relapses and remissions. About 65 percent of patients initially suffer from relapsing-remitting MS, and about 40 percent shift to secondary progressive MS, usually over a period of 15 to 20 years. Approximately 350,000 people have been diagnosed with MS in the United States, with an estimated 10,000 new cases diagnosed annually. Most people with MS experience their first symptoms and are diagnosed between the ages of 15 and 50. A woman is three times more likely to develop MS than a man. Symptoms are often accompanied by extreme fatigue and heat intolerance.

Presently, there is no cure for MS. Current medications aim to slow the disease progression, reducing the frequency and severity of attacks and the development of new brain lesions. These drugs, termed immune system modulators, include three varieties of interferon and two other similar-acting agents, all of which need to be injected on a continuous basis. A small, seven-patient NIH clinical trial using recombinant Insulin-Like Growth Factor-1 (rhIGF-1) did not show statistically significant improvement, but the popular conception is that a combination of growth factor therapies may prove to be more promising.

CVBT will begin its animal testing phase for Parkinson's disease, ALS, and Multiple Sclerosis in 2005.

27: Outlook

Perfusion and oxygen supply are the most critical issues for living tissues and organs. Because every living cell needs oxygen to survive, the "pathway system" – i.e., the arteries, arterioles, capillaries, and the venous system – and their regular function is essential to the human body. Most ischemic tissues are generally unable to mount an adequate physiological response to reverse disease processes, particularly hypoxia and ischemia. Patients with advanced Coronary Artery Disease often have insufficient collateralization to prevent ischemic damage and, barring medical or surgical intervention, eventual infarction. Acute stroke patients are unable to generate sufficient neo-vascularization to salvage ischemic brain tissue and prevent the loss of neurological function. Patients with end-stage Peripheral Vascular Disease suffer from critical limb ischemia and are unable to induce sufficient angiogenesis to reverse skin ulceration and gangrene. Patients with chronic wound ischemia lack the appropriate angiogenic response to generate granulation tissue for complete wound healing.

Our basic research and our clinical trials with humans have taught us the impressive power borne by FGF-1 in initiating the process of angiogenesis in hypoxic or ischemic tissues. We have also learned that there are no serious side effects, and particularly no risk of tumour growth or generation. It has been demonstrated that in Coronary Heart Disease, the efficacy of an intramyocardial treatment with FGF-1 is a reality. Because of its diverse powers in the art of tissue repair, FGF-1 might become one of the most groundbreaking drugs in the fight against many different diseases – all of them dependant on its ability to ...

- initiate neoangiogenesis,
- repair and protect nerve tissue and neurons,
- and repair and protect cartilage tissue.

Thus, all diseases characterized by a lack of perfusion – hypoxia, ischemia – are potential candidates for a FGF-1 treatment – independent of the individual organ or tissue in the human body. Such diseases include:

- Coronary Heart Disease
- Ischemic Cardiomyopathy
- Transplant Vasculopathy
- Cerebrovascular Disease
- Peripheral Vascular Disease
- Protecting Surgical Anastomoses
- Wounds
- Skin Ulcers
- Lumbar Ischemia

In addition, various *cerebral diseases* may be treated by FGF-1 – particularly when the dependent tissues require improved perfusion and blood supply.

Also, a combination of stem cell therapy and FGF-1-therapy (i.e., replacing/regenerating myocardial cells *and* providing the perfusion and oxygen supply) might emerge as an indication for patients suffering from terminal cardiomyopathy *not* caused by Coronary Artery Disease (so-called "Dilatative Cardiomyopathy").

Finally, degenerative or infective diseases involving the cartilage of any articulation (Articular Rheumatism, for example) may well become entities for which FGF-1 is a new treatment option.

A great deal of research still begs to be conducted. Shall we get on with it? The story of therapeutic angiogenesis is a massive epic, and I'm pleased to report that it has only just begun.

References (Selected):

1. Schumacher, B, Pecher, P, von Specht, BU, & Stegmann,TJ:
   Induction of Neoangiogenesis in Ischemic Myocardium by
   Human Growth Factors. First Clinical Results of a New Treatment
   of Coronary Heart Disease.

   Circulation 97: 645-650 (1998)

2. Stegmann, TJ:
   FGF-1: A human growth factor in the induction of neoangiogenesis.

   Exp.Opin.Invest.Drugs 7: 2011-2015 (1998)

3. Schumacher, B, Stegmann,TJ, & Pecher, P:
   The stimulation of neoangiogenesis in the ischemic human
   heart by the growth factor FGF: First clinical results.

   J.Cardiovasc.Surg. 39: 783-789 (1998)

4. Stegmann, TJ:
   New Approaches to Coronary Heart Disease.
   Induction of Neovascularization by Growth Factors.

   BioDrugs 11: 301-308 (1999)

5. Stegmann,TJ, Hoppert, T:
   Combined Local Angiogenesis and Surgical
   Revascularization for Coronary Heart Disease.

   Current Intervent.Cardiol.Reports 1: 172-178 (1999)

6. Stegmann, TJ:
   Intramyocardial injection of acidic fibroblast growth factor: adjunct
   to bypass surgery and monotherapy for coronary heart disease.

   In: Handbook of Myocardial Revascularization and Angiogenesis, ed. R.
   Kornosky, S.E. Epstein, M. Leon. M. Dunitz Ltd., London, 1999, p.201-214.

7. Stegmann, TJ:
   Myocardial Neo-Angiogenesis by Local Application of Growth Factors

   In: XXI Congress of the Europ.Soc.Cardiology, ed. F.Navarro-Lopez.
   Monduzzi Editore, Internat.Proceedings Division, Bologna, Italy, 1999, p.319-322.

8. Stegmann, TJ, Hoppert, T, Schlürmann, W, & Gemeinhardt, S:
   First Angiogenic Treatment of Coronary Heart Disease by FGF 1:
   Long-Term Results after 3 Years.

   CVR 1: 5-10 (2000)

9. Stegmann, TJ, Hoppert, T:
    Gentherapie bei kardiovaskulären Erkrankungen.

    J.Kardiol. 7: 292-295 (2000)

10. Stegmann,TJ, Hoppert,T, Schneider, A, Gemeinhardt, S, Köcher, M,
    Ibing, R, & Strupp, G:
    Induktion der myokardialen Neoangiogenese durch humane
    Wachstumsfaktoren. Ein neuer Therapieansatz bei koronarer Herzkrankheit.

    Herz 25: 589-599 (2000)

11. Stegmann, TJ:
    New Approaches to Coronary Heart Disease. Induction of Neovascularization
    by Growth Factors.

    In: Preventing Coronary Heart Disease, ed. A.Prakash. Adis
    Internat. Limited, Auckland-Madrid-Philadelphia, 2000, p.79-86.

12. Simons, M, Bonow, RO, Chronos, NA, Cohen, DJ, Giordano, FJ, Hammond, HK,
    Laham, RJ, Li, W, Pike, M, Sellke, FW, Stegmann, TJ, Udelson, JE,
    & Rosengart, TK:
    Clinical Trials in Coronary Angiogenesis: Issues, Problems, Consensus.

    Circulation 102: e73-e86 (2000)

13. Hoppert, T, Ibing, R, Schneider, A, Popp, M, & Stegmann, TJ:
    Klinische Ergebnisse der Behandlung der koronaren
    Herzkrankheit mit Wachstumsfaktoren.

    Hämostaseologie 20: 167-172 (2000)

14. Wagoner, L.E., Snavely, D.D., Conway, G.A., Hauntz, E.A., &
    Merrill, W.H.:
    Intramyocardial Injection of Fibroblast Growth Factor-1 for
    Treatment of Refractory Angina Pectoris: The Initial US Experience.

    Circulation 110, Suppl. III, 395 (2004)

"For one human being to love another:
that is perhaps the most difficult of our tasks;
the ultimate, the last test and proof,
the work for which all other work is but preparation."

RAINER MARIA RILKE, 1875–1926
GERMAN LYRIC POET

Biography

Thomas J. Stegmann, M.D., Prof. of Surgery

Dr. Thomas J. Stegmann is a Cardiovascular Surgeon, Professor of Surgery, and the Director of the Department for Thoracic & Cardiovascular Surgery at the Fulda Medical Center, Fulda, Germany. The Fulda Medical Center is a major medical and teaching hospital serving the University of Marburg and the greater Frankfurt, Germany, area. Dr. Stegmann is also a Member of the Faculty of the Hannover Medical School, Germany.

Dr. Stegmann is also a medical research scientist, who has been working the last 10 years on the area of Neo-Angiogenesis and Human Growth Factors. His medical research work has lead to the discovery of a way of stimulating the growth of new blood vessels in the human heart, which can be used in the treatment for the heart disease commonly known as coronary artery (heart) disease (or clogged heart arteries). Coronary heart disease is the leading cause of death in the developed world. It is a reported and well-known fact that 50% of all people in the developed world die of coronary heart disease. Dr. Stegmann's discovery opens a new area of biotechnology and medical treatment for the treatment of this disease.

Dr. Stegmann is co-editor of the journal "Cardiac and Vascular Regeneration". He is also a Member of the Faculty of "Trans-Catheter Therapeutics", Cardiovascular Research Foundation (CRF) of the United States (New York).

Dr. Stegmann has written numerous articles (more than 200) for medical scientific publications, including the world famous scientific journal "Circulation", which is published by the American Heart Association.

Dr. Stegmann is a Founder and Director of Cardio Vascular Bio Therapeutics Inc., a United States biotechnology company, which is commercialising Dr. Stegmann's medical discovery to treat heart disease, and peripheral atherosclerotic disease.

Dr. Stegmann is a speaker of world repute in the fields of biotechnology, medical research and cardiovascular diseases.

Dr. Thomas (Joseph) Stegmann

Thomas J. Stegmann, M.D., Prof. of Surgery, Director of the Department of Thoracic and Cardiovascular Surgery, Fulda Medical Center, Germany.

Curriculum vitae

11-20-1946	Born as the son of Adalbert Stegmann and his wife Marianne in Hannover, Germany.
1953-1957	Attending primary school in Hannover and Bad Godesberg/Bonn, Germany.
1957-1966	Attending High School (Gymnasium), „Aloisius-Kolleg"- Classical education with modern linguistic section.
2-24-1966	Baccalaureate (Abitur).
1966-1967	Immatriculated at the Faculty of Philosophy at Munich and Bonn University, Germany: Studies of German Literature, Philosophy, and History.
1968	Changed to the Faculty of Medicine at Bonn University and commenced with studies of Human Medicine.
10-13-1969	Preexamen of Natural Science (**Grade A**).
03-03-1971	Preexamen of Medicine (**Grade A**).

06-28-1974   Final examination (**Grade A**) after 6 semesters of
              medicine at Heidelberg University.

07-01-1974   Doctor thesis (**summa cum laude**):
              Catecholamingehalt und Enzymaktivitaetsveraende
              rungen des Herzmuskels bei tierexperimenteller
              Herzhypertrophie (Content of Catecholamines
              and Change in Enzyme-Activities of the
              Cardiac Muscle in Experimentally
              Hypertrophied Hearts)

Awarded by Price of Faculty for the **Best Dissertation**
of the Medical Faculty of the University of Heidelberg.

1974-1976   Pre-clinical training in Surgery and Internal Medicine.

08-01-1975   Certified Medical Doctor (Approbation).

1976-1982   Fellow at the Department of Surgery,
              Hannover Medical School (Prof. Dr. Hans G. **Borst**).

During this time, spent 12 months at the Division of Traumatology
(Prof. Dr. Harald **Tscherne**) and 18 months at the Division of
Abdominal and Transplant Surgery (Prof. Dr. Rudolf **Pichlmayr**).

01-22-1982   „Facharzt fuer Chirurgie"
              (Aerztekammer Niedersachsen).

02-19-1982   Awarded the „**Rudolf - Nissen - Memorial - Price**"
              by the Deutsche Gesellschaft fuer

Thorax-, Herz und Gefaesschirurgie
(German Society for Thoracic
and Cardiovascular Surgery).

07-07-1982   Docent thesis (venia legendi in surgery):
„Die systemische Luftembolie. Experimentelle
Untersuchungen zur koronaren undcerebralen
Luftembolie" (Systemic air embolism).

1982-1985   Resident at the Division of Thoracic and Cardiovascular
Surgery (Prof. Dr. Hans G. **Borst**), **Hannover Medical
School**, Germany.

11-10-1983   Teilgebietsbezeichnungen „Thorax- und Kardiovaskul
archirurgie" und „Gefaesschirurgie"
(Aerztekammer Niedersachsen).

07-12-1989   Appointment to **Professor of Surgery**,
Hannover Medical School.

Since 01-01-1985

Director of the Department for Thoracic and Cardiovascular Surgery,
Fulda Medical Center, Germany (Teaching Hospital, University
of Marburg, Germany) and **Member of the Faculty of Hannover
Medical School.** Stress points of clinical and scientific work: coronary
surgery, surgery for aortic diseases (especially aortic dissection), heart
valve surgery, heart transplantation, lung transplantation, vascular
surgery, pacemaker-and-AICD-surgery, surgery of the oesophagus,
neo-angiogenesis, and human growth factors.